PROFESSIONAL HEALTH REGULATION IN THE PUBLIC INTEREST

International perspectives

Edited by
John Martyn Chamberlain, Mike Dent and Mike Saks

First published in Great Britain in 2018 by

Policy Press
University of Bristol
1-9 Old Park Hill
Bristol
BS2 8BB
UK
t: +44 (0)117 954 5940
pp-info@bristol.ac.uk
www.policypress.co.uk

North America office:
Policy Press
c/o The University of Chicago Press
1427 East 60th Street
Chicago, IL 60637, USA
t: +1 773 702 7700
f: +1 773-702-9756
sales@press.uchicago.edu
www.press.uchicago.edu

© Policy Press 2018

British Library Cataloguing in Publication Data
A catalogue record for this book is available from the British Library

Library of Congress Cataloging-in-Publication Data
A catalog record for this book has been requested

ISBN 978-1-4473-3226-8 hardcover
ISBN 978-1-4473-3533-7 ePub
ISBN 978-1-4473-3534-4 Mobi
ISBN 978-1-4473-3227-5 ePdf

The right of John Martyn Chamberlain, Mike Dent and Mike Saks to be identified as editors of this work has been asserted by them in accordance with the Copyright, Designs and Patents Act 1988.

The statements and opinions contained within this publication are solely those of the editors and contributors and not of the University of Bristol or Policy Press. The University of Bristol and Policy Press disclaim responsibility for any injury to persons or property resulting from any material published in this publication.

Policy Press works to counter discrimination on grounds of gender, race, disability, age and sexuality.

Cover design by Qube Design Associates, Bristol
Front cover image: istock
Printed and bound in Great Britain by CPI Group (UK) Ltd, Croydon, CR0 4YY
Policy Press uses environmentally responsible print partners

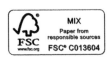

Contents

List of tables

Notes on contributors

Humayun Ahmed is a Research Assistant in Health Policy and an MSc candidate in the Institute of Medical Science at the University of Toronto, Canada. His research interests involve international health policy, genetics and epidemiology. He is also engaged in compliance research, teaching and education entrepreneurship.

Judith Allsop is a Visiting Professor in the School of Health and Social Care at the University of Lincoln and Professor Emerita at London South Bank University, UK. Drawing on the disciplines of both social policy and the sociology of health and illness, she has researched and published books and articles on health policy, complaints and user involvement in health care settings and the regulation of health professionals. A third edition of a jointly edited book with Mike Saks on *Researching Health: Qualitative, Quantitative and Mixed Methods* (2019) is in progress. She has served on a number of UK government committees and local health management boards.

Joana Almeida is a sociologist with research interests in the sociology of health, illness and the professions. She is Lecturer in Applied Social Studies at the University of Bedfordshire, having previously been a Teaching Fellow in Sociology in the School of Law at Royal Holloway, University of London, UK. She recently held a Postdoctoral Research Fellow funded by the Foundation for the Sociology of Health and Illness. Her publications have appeared in journals such as *Health* and *Social Science and Medicine*.

Nelson Barros is a social scientist with research interests in the sociology of health, illness and care. He is an Associate Professor in the Faculty of Medical Sciences at the University of Campinas, Brazil. He is the long-term coordinator of the Brazilian Laboratory for Alternative, Complementary and Integrative Health Practices (LAPACIS). He has been a Visiting Scholar at the University of Leeds (2006–08) and at the University of London (2017), UK. He has published extensively in academic journals and edited books and is the author of various books on qualitative health research.

Marie Bismark is a public health physician, health lawyer and company director. She works in the Law and Public Health Unit at the Melbourne School of Population and Global Health, Australia. She previously served as a legal adviser to the New Zealand Health and Disability Commissioner and completed a Harkness Fellowship in Healthcare Policy at Harvard University, United States. Her research focuses on the role of clinical governance, regulation and patient complaints in improving the quality and safety of health care.

Adalsteinn Brown is the Interim Dean of the Dalla Lana School of Public Health and the Dalla Lana Chair of Public Health Policy at the University of Toronto, Canada. Previously he was the head of strategy and policy for the Ontario Ministry of Health and Long-Term Care and for science and research at the Ontario Ministry of Research and Innovation. His public service and academic career has focused heavily around issues of quality improvement and evidence use. He is a graduate of Harvard and Oxford Universities.

Patrick Brown is an Associate Professor in the Department of Sociology at the University of Amsterdam, The Netherlands. His research explores trust, risk, hope and related social processes by which individuals, professional groups and organisations cope amid uncertainty, especially in health care contexts. His recent books include *Trusting on the Edge* (2012) with Michael Calnan, *Making Health Policy: A Critical Introduction* (2012) with Andy Alaszewski, and the edited volume *Theories of Uncertainty and Risk across Different Modernities* (2018). His immersion within Amsterdam sociology has led to a growing interest in Eliasian analyses.

Michael Calnan is a Professor of Medical Sociology in the School of Social Policy, Sociology and Social Research at the University of Kent, UK. He is a medical sociologist and has researched and published extensively on a wide range of health-related topics. His books include *Health, Medicine and Society: Key Theories, Future Agendas* (2000), *Work Stress: The Making of a Modern Epidemic* (2002), *Trust Matters in Health Care* (2008), *The New Sociology of the Health Service* (2009) and *Trusting on the Edge* (2012). His current research includes a sociological study of the recent Ebola epidemic in West Africa.

John Martyn Chamberlain is Professor of Criminology and Public Policy at Swansea University. His concerns with governance and regulation are multidisciplinary, covering socio-legal studies, philosophy, ethics, statistics and machine learning. His books include *Doctoring Medical Governance: Medical Self-Regulation in Transition* (2009), *Medical Regulation: An Introduction* (2013), *Medical Regulation, Fitness to Practice and Medical Revalidation* (2015) and *Medicine, Risk, Discourse and Power* (2016). He is currently conducting research into the role of disruptive digital technologies, Bayesian statistics and artificial intelligence with the

Professional Standards Authority and all nine UK Professional Regulators it oversees. Additionally, he is writing a book entitled *Healthcare Governance and Disruptive Regulatory Algorithms: The Role of Machine Learning and Artificial Intelligence* which will be published in late 2018.

Mike Dent is an Emeritus Professor at Staffordshire University and Visiting Professor at Leicester University, UK. He continues to research and publish on the professions, especially on the comparative study of the professions and management within health care organisations, as well as user and citizen involvement in its various forms. His most recent book is entitled *The Routledge Companion to the Professions and Professionalism* (2016) and he has contributed a number of chapters on related topics. His articles have appeared in a range of leading academic journals, including *Public Administration, Organization, Organizational Studies* and *Sociology of Health and Illness.*

Rubén Flores is Assistant Professor of Sociology at the Higher School of Economics in Moscow, Russia. He is also a Visiting Lecturer at University College Dublin School of Sociology and a Visiting Scholar at Maynooth University Department of Sociology, Ireland. His fields of interest include the study of compassion and care (especially in health care contexts), medical humanities, and the dialogue between Buddhism and social research.

Ruth Horowitz is a Professor of Sociology at New York University, United States. Among her books are *Honor and the American Dream: Culture and Identity in a Chicano Community* (1983), *Teen Mothers, Citizens or Dependents?* (1995) and *In the Public Interest: Medical Licensing and the Disciplinary Process* (2013). Currently, she serves as a public member on the boards of three medical organisations. Her latest research focuses on ballet careers and labour markets.

Kathryn Jones is a Senior Research Fellow at De Montfort University, UK. She is based in the Department of Politics and Public Policy and is a member of the Health Policy Research Unit (HPRU), a cross-disciplinary group of researchers. She has published extensively in academic journals, including *Policy and Politics, Social Science and Medicine* and *Sociology of Health and Illness.* Her main research interests are patient and public involvement, health system reform, health professional regulation and the links between patients' organisations and the pharmaceutical industry.

Sumit Kane is a Senior Research Fellow at the Nossal Institute for Global Health, University of Melbourne, Australia, and a Visiting Professor at the Gokhale Institute of Politics and Economics, Pune, India. He is a medical doctor who has researched and published extensively on a wide range of topics in global health research, policy and practice. In his work he examines issues from multiple perspectives – social, cultural and operational – to inform the development of feasible solutions in different contexts.

Jennifer Moore is a Senior Lecturer at the University of New South Wales, Australia, and a barrister and solicitor of the New Zealand High Court. She was the 2015–16 New Zealand Harkness Fellow in Healthcare Policy at Stanford University, United States. She previously served as a legal adviser to the New Zealand Law Commissioners. She was also Senior Lecturer in Preventive Medicine and Acting Director of the Legal Issues Centre at the University of Otago, New Zealand, and Lecturer in Health Sciences at Monash University, Australia. Her research and teaching expertise is in health law, coronial law, torts, law and technology, and empirical legal research methods.

Jennifer Morris is a Researcher in the School of Population and Global Health at the University of Melbourne, Australia. She is a health care quality and safety researcher, health care consumer representative and science communicator. She also holds several governance and advisory positions, including being a member of the Victorian Clinical Council, Better Care Victoria and the Victorian Disability Advisory Council, Department of Health and Human Services. Prior to joining the University of Melbourne, she was a Research Officer at Young and Well Cooperative Research Centre and a science communicator at the Murdoch Children's Research Institute.

Fiona Pacey is a PhD candidate at the University of Sydney, Australia. Her research is examining the creation of the National Registration and Accreditation Scheme for the Health Professions in Australia and its accountability framework, drawing on her interests in Australia's federal system of government and health workforce policy and strategy. She has worked in policy and management roles in the field of medical education for over 15 years.

William Roche is Professor of Pathology at the University of Southampton, UK. He chairs the Wessex Clinical Senate, advising and assuring major changes in health care provision and is a senior appraiser for NHS England South, conducting annual appraisals of Medical Directors and Responsible Officers. His previous roles include Medical Director of

NHS South East Coast Strategic Health Authority and Medical Director and Deputy Chief Executive of Southampton University Hospitals NHS Trust. He is a Founding Senior Fellow of the Faculty of Medical Leadership and Management.

Mike Saks is Emeritus Professor at the University of Suffolk and Visiting Professor at the University of Lincoln, Plymouth Marjon University, and the Royal Veterinary College, the University of London, all in the UK, and the University of Toronto, Canada. He has served on the executive/boards of six universities, including as Chief Executive, and has acted as a chair/member of NHS committees at all levels. He has also been an adviser to governments and professional bodies internationally in health and social care and has made many keynote presentations at conferences – having published numerous articles and book chapters and over 15 books in his specialist areas of health, the professions and regulation from a social science perspective.

Stephanie Short leads Workforce Development Activities in the World Health Organization (WHO) Collaborating Centre in Health Workforce Development in Rehabilitation and Long Term Care, Australia. She is Deputy Director of the Sydney University Asia Pacific Migration Centre, Australia, and is Academic Lead of the Shaping Health Systems Research Group, World Universities Network. She has published widely in health sociology and public policy, including *Health Workforce Governance* (2012) as co-editor, and the fifth edition of *Health Care and Public Policy: An Australian Analysis* (2014) as co-author.

Pâmela Siegel is a Brazilian psychologist. She has been active in the third sector and is a specialist in analytical psychology. Her main field of interest is the interface between psychology, religion and health. Her main studies have focused on yoga and on the use of acupuncture, medicinal herbs and reiki by cancer patients. She is currently a member of the Laboratory for Alternative, Complementary and Integrative Health Practices (LAPACIS) at the University of Campinas, Brazil.

Karsten Vrangbæk is a Professor in the Department of Political Science and the Department of Public Health at the University of Copenhagen, Denmark. He is Head of the Centre for Health Economics and Policy (CHEP) and theme leader in the Centre for Healthy Ageing (CEHA) at the same university. His research interests include comparative health policy, public administration and management, organisation and the evaluation of health care. He has published extensively on these issues in international journals and books.

Foreword

Richard B. Saltman

The structure of professional regulation in health care emerged as an important policy issue in the early 1990s. The initial discussion of regulatory reform had already begun a decade earlier at the more general policy level in many countries (Baldwin et al, 1998). Subsequently, in the health sector, once previously in lockstep, publicly administered hospitals in many Western and Central European countries were transformed into varying degrees of semi-autonomous and/or self-managing organisations (Saltman et al, 2011). Responding to this change, governments introduced revised regulatory arrangements through which to supervise provider behaviour and ensure clinically, financially and socially satisfactory outcomes. These new institutional and regulatory arrangements were conjoined at the popular level with increased patient pressure in a number of tax-funded health systems for reductions in waiting lists, as well as increased choice of health care provider and/or provider institution (Saltman and von Otter, 1992; Le Grand and Bartlett, 1993). In the first decade of the 2000s, reflecting this newly diverse service delivery environment, concepts such as 'stewardship' and 'governance' began to receive attention in policymaking circles (Saltman and Ferroussier-Davis, 2000; Saltman et al, 2011), and in a number of country contexts, existing regulatory measures were further re-thought, re-justified and (depending on the country) reconfigured.

While the overall purpose and function of health sector regulation remained largely constant, the process and mechanisms through which regulation acted was changed, in some cases quite considerably (Osborne and Gaebler, 1992; Kettl, 1993). Regulation became a more extensive, diverse and complex endeavour, expanding its scope and focus in a variety of different national contexts. In addition to redesigned efforts at national level, varying degrees of de-concentration (independent national agencies), delegation (private organisations) and devolution (regional and local governments) were brought into play. In England, different national agencies – with various degrees of independent structure – were introduced in succession (Saltman, 2012). In Sweden, new supervisory efforts in the 1990s by the National Board of Health and Welfare were supplemented in 2006 by the introduction of 'open comparisons', by which the Ministry of Social

Affairs and Health published performance measures of each regional public delivery agency (with 21 elected county and regional councils). Similarly, but somewhat less successfully, Italy in 1999 and Spain in 2003 introduced national arrangements to monitor service quality and outcomes among their public regional health care providers.

After 2008, with the onset of the global financial crisis, the complexity of the health sector regulatory process increased notably. Substantially reduced public revenues and the start of a decade of continued fiscal austerity across most publicly funded health systems, as well as the rapid introduction of new information technologies in medicine and management, meant that the mechanisms of regulation in the health sector had to become more agile and better targeted. The accompanying, sometimes dramatic, increase in new clinical technologies in the health sector, driven at the international level by private providers in largely privately funded health systems in economically stronger countries such as Switzerland and the United States, put further pressure on both the regulatory process in publicly funded systems – to match clinical possibilities and outcomes – as well as the previously adopted national patient treatment guarantees (in Denmark, England, Norway and Sweden, among others) that had been introduced in response to patient pressure for reduced waiting times. Regulatory ruptures such as that which occurred at the beginning of this new period of fiscal austerity at Mid Staffordshire NHS Foundation Trust in England further compounded the political pressure on national authorities.

In the new policy environment that has emerged post-crisis, regulation going forward will need to respond to an increasingly diverse and also disrupted health care delivery environments. Organisationally, public hospitals and health centres in many publicly funded health systems in Europe and beyond face considerable pressure from rapidly growing private systems of providers. Clinically, a generational shift in medical technology tied to each patient's genome and the ensuing demand for 'personal medicine' – as well as technologically driven capacities for patient self-monitoring and co-production in their homes – will test the ability of regulators to encourage new delivery approaches, while maintaining adequate purview over quality and outcomes. More broadly, the development of integrated networks of care for the growing population of chronically ill older people will force regulators to rethink many of the intermediate targets and mechanisms that particularly professional regulation has required.

These and other associated technological changes will force regulators to consider how health sector regulation can be again reshaped to become less a part of the (static) problem and more a part of the (dynamic) solution that contemporary health care systems now require (Jeurissen et al, 2016).

The current volume provides insights into a wide range of regulatory concepts, experiences and possibilities across a range of advanced and – with Brazil, India and Russia – middle-income countries. Individual chapters review important regulatory initiatives in leading countries such as England, Sweden and the United States, as well as Australia and Canada. Drawing on contributors from a wide range of academic disciplines, including political science, sociology and medicine, many with direct experience in national and international organisations, the chapters present a timely assessment of the current state of regulatory thinking about health care professionals, and a set of useful guideposts for future policy debate and decision making. The book will certainly play an important role in what will be a central issue in improving the overall effectiveness of health systems in coming years.

References

Baldwin, R, Scott, C. and Hood, C. (eds) (1998) *A Reader on Regulation*, Oxford: Oxford University Press.

Jeurissen, P., Duran, A. and Saltman, R. B. (2016) 'Uncomfortable realities: the challenge of making real change inside Europe's consolidating hospital sector', *BMC Health Services Research*, 16(suppl 2): 168.

Kettl, D. (1993) *Sharing Power*, Washington, DC: Brookings Institution.

Le Grand, J. and Bartlett, W. (1993) *Quasi-Markets and Public Policy*, London: Macmillan.

Osborne, D. and Gaebler, T. (1992) *Re-Inventing Government*, Reading, MA: Addison-Wesley.

Saltman, R. B. (2012) 'The role of regulation in healthcare', *British Medical Journal* 344: e821.

Saltman, R. B., Duran, A. and Dubois, H. W. F. (eds) (2011) *Governing Public Hospitals: Recent Strategies and the Movement Toward Institutional Autonomy*, Brussels: European Observatory on Health Systems and Policies.

Saltman, R. B. and Ferroussier-Davis, O. (2000) 'The concept of stewardship in health policy', *Bulletin of the World Health Organization/ International Journal of Public Health* 78(June): 732-39.

Saltman, R. B. and von Otter, C. (1992) *Planned Markets and Public Competition: Strategic Reform in Northern European Health Systems*, Buckingham: Open University Press.

Editors' overview

This volume is the first in a series entitled the *Sociology of Health Professions: Future International Directions*, published by Policy Press and edited by Mike Saks and Mike Dent, supported by a high-profile international advisory board. The research-based series is focused on giving innovatory sociological insights into the past, present and future development of the health professions. It is primarily oriented towards final-year and postgraduate students, academic lecturers/researchers, practitioners and policy makers. Its general aims are:

- to inform and stimulate debate about issues in the sociology of health professions;
- to influence policy development and practice in the fields concerned;
- to make a significant contribution to academic thinking in the sociology of health; and
- to produce original national/international work of recognised high quality.

This present volume on *Professional Health Regulation in the Public Interest: International Perspectives* is the first to be published under the series banner. Its significance in terms of the series is underlined by the positive contextual words in the Foreword by a world-renowned academic leader in the field of comparative health policy, Richard B. Saltman. It is co-edited by John Martyn Chamberlain, Mike Dent and Mike Saks – the first of whom introduces the volume and its various contributions in the initial chapter of this flagship book. It is anticipated that the book will fill an important gap in the literature, drawing on the strongest work internationally on the regulation of health professions. This edited collection is also characterised by its breadth of coverage of health professional groups and the depth of knowledge and experience of its contributors in combining academically rigorous analysis with a policy thrust. As such, it should appeal not only to academics and practitioners, but also to regulators – including government policy makers and professional bodies themselves. This policy orientation and a focus on positive socio-political impact will continue to be the kitemark of other books in the series as it moves forward over the coming years, with the backing of Policy Press.

Mike Saks and Mike Dent

ONE

Introduction: professional health regulation in the public interest

John Martyn Chamberlain

Health care regulation: some global trends

This timely volume focuses on the regulation of professional groups involved in the delivery of health services internationally. In so doing, it brings together leading authors from Australasia, Europe, India, North and South America and Russia who share a concern with how occupations with highly specialist forms of expertise are regulated, the role that members of the public play within this and, relatedly, whose interests are best served by the arrangements in place. Indeed, it is important to highlight a core common theme that underpins the chapters presented here – namely, that it is possible to ascertain from an international perspective that the academic analysis of the professions and their regulation is gradually moving away from solely focusing on advocating greater 'outsider' involvement in the regulation of occupations classified as professions, towards also recognising the need to capture and critically scrutinise what exactly is meant by the term 'public interest'. Therefore, it is necessary to first provide some conceptual background on current developments globally in the regulation of health care practitioners, before moving on to introduce the contributions that follow in subsequent chapters.

It is necessary to begin by stating unequivocally that how professional groups are regulated varies considerably across international jurisdictions, as the chapters in this volume illustrate. Nonetheless, it is possible to discern, albeit in the broadest of brushstrokes, important similarities between countries worldwide (Giarelli et al, 2014). Certainly, rising running costs associated with the delivery of increasingly complex health and social care services, have led countries as diverse as China, India, Japan, Russia and the United States (US) to act in the past two decades to embed non-medical involvement in the delivery of health care services and their quality assurance (Bismark et al, 2015; Pan et al, 2015; Saks, 2015; Toth, 2015; Walton-Roberts, 2015). Although significant national variation exists in how this state of affairs both presents itself and plays out, the key result, particularly in Western nation states, has been an intensification and expansion of bureaucratic and managerial discourses and practices shaping the activity of the health care system and monitoring the performance of professional work (de Vries et al, 2009; Risso-Gill et al, 2014). Recent developments in neural-net computing, big data and artificial intelligence technologies will undoubtedly in the coming decades take this unfolding administrative and managerial landscape in new and unforeseen directions, as their use as diagnostic and predictive tools to help reduce medical errors and costs – as well as to promote public health and patient safety – becomes ever more apparent (Altman, 2017; Miotto et al, 2017). But, for now, what is clear is that professional groups no longer possess the degree of occupational control and autonomy over the generation and application of their technical skill as they perhaps once did, particularly in the Anglo-American, Australasian and pan-European contexts (Chamberlain, 2015). This is a point this chapter will return to shortly.

The value of patients for ensuring the more effective management of health care costs and risks has also become an essential part of the international contemporary regulatory reform and performance management agenda, and this role can likewise be expected to increase – as well as take hitherto unexpected directions – in the coming decades (Giarelli et al, 2014). This said, it is already clear that a key emergent factor that needs to be addressed at policy and practice levels is the limited conception of public involvement that can be found in the Australasian, European and US contexts in particular. Indeed, many informed contributors suggest that patient involvement in regulatory regimes tends to be limited to particular elite interest groups, rather than reflecting broader social strata in these diverse societies (McDonald, 2012; Chadderton et al, 2013; Beaupert et al, 2014; Bismark et al, 2015; Saks, 2015). For example, Bouwman and colleagues (2015) concluded, after reviewing the Dutch regulatory system, that enhanced practitioner accountability and improvement in the detection of problems in health care will only emerge when a long-term learning commitment is made, on behalf of government and professional groups, to promote more expansive and inclusive public participation mechanisms. However, a key issue here is that the academic regulatory literature has perhaps been too focused on promoting public involvement in health care regulation at the cost of more fully reflecting on what is meant by the contested term 'public interest' in the context of the regulation of professional groups (Saks, 1995). It is important that we do not define the public interest solely in terms of the degree and nature of public involvement in health care quality assurance processes and the regulation of professional work. Indeed, a shared preoccupation with unpacking the complex relationships that exist between promoting greater 'public involvement' in health care and advocating the 'public interest', is present in all of the following chapters. However, before this is discussed further, it is first necessary to briefly examine current academic discourse surrounding the regulation of the professions.

The sociology of the professions: a cautionary tale

In the preceding section, it was noted that it is a common contemporary trend internationally that a traditional core feature of professional occupations such as medicine – including the technical expertise involved – has become increasingly subject to third-party scrutiny and control (Chamberlain, 2017b). Yet this is not a new trend; sociologists interested in the professions have been highlighting since the late 1970s that the openness of modern health care to codification and rationalisation – often in the form of the generation of best-evidence guidance and practice-based protocols – carried with it the danger of making its underpinning specialist technical expertise increasingly more open to third-party scrutiny and administrative performance management (Chamberlain, 2015). This trend arguably was in tension with the dominant 'social closure' model of professional regulation present in the literature on the sociology of the professions (Chamberlain, 2012). In this model, fledging occupational groups attempt to use their esoteric technical expertise to claim professional standing by claiming to use it in the service of the public good rather than solely for pecuniary gain (Freidson, 2001). The goal over time is to persuade the governing state to create legislative enclosures around their activities, which in turn enables them to exclude non-members from entry, training, discipline and exit arrangements (Allsop and Saks, 2002).

Although clearly a high-level abstraction of real-world historical events, this model served Anglo-American and European academics in particular relatively well as a tool for unpacking the complex relationships that existed from the 19th century onwards between the state, civil society and occupations successfully classified as professions (Barry et al, 2013). As a result, the tension over time between this model and the unfolding events relating to the increasing codification and external scrutiny of professional forms of technical expertise has meant that it has been subject to a degree of refinement (Chamberlain, 2012). So rather than being held to possess a modicum of absolute control and autonomy over their training, work and disciplinary activities, professional groups are now held to possess a form of devolved or regulated autonomy (Freidson, 2001). Later in this volume, Judith Allsop and Kathryn Jones provide a ready example of such unfolding developments in the United Kingdom (UK) when they discuss the emergence of the meta-regulator, the Professional Standards Authority, to oversee the work of traditionally autonomous professional health care regulators such as the General Medical Council (GMC).

A key aspect of the utility of the 'social closure' model is its ability to provide a historical grounded framework from which it was possible to track contemporary developments in the regulation of the medical profession in the Anglo-American context in particular. However, there was a growing concern in some quarters from the early 1990s onwards that the public interest tended to be conceptualised within the sociological literature concerned with the professions as if it was cynically bartered by occupational groups as part of their strategy to obtain, and maintain, their professional status (Chamberlain, 2012). Indeed, although the sociological analysis of professional groups in its early stages perhaps was too ready to accept the public avowal of 'do no harm' espoused by occupations such as medicine, the latter cynicism of the moral basis of the professional project pursued by such occupations was perhaps a little exaggerated (Stacey, 1992). Certainly, a fierce commitment to the ideal of public service by practitioners is a common feature of many accounts of their experiences and perceptions of regulatory reforms over the past two decades (Chamberlain, 2015) – albeit in the US the focus of medical professional ethics is more on serving the client than the collective good that is emphasised in Britain (Saks, 2015).

Freidson (2001) and Stacey (1992, 2000) both argued that adopting a cynical attitude towards the 'virtue ethics' that underpin the profession of medicine obfuscates further the complex problem of 'how to [both] nurture and control occupations with complex, esoteric knowledge and skill … which provide us with critical personal services' (Freidson, 2001: 220). This conclusion is also grounded in the recognition that the changing nature of professional regulation is not solely (or indeed primarily) a response to a series of high-profile scandals, such as the mass murderer and general practitioner Harold Shipman in the UK. Rather, it is bound up with broader shifts in contemporary styles of governance that are aimed at transforming the ways in which states engage with their subject-citizens as much as they are concerned with the ways in which the professions manage their affairs (Chamberlain, 2012). In other words, contemporary reforms in professional regulation can be said to also be bound up with a broader shift in the conditions under which 'good governance' can be seen to be legitimately practised – especially in liberal democratic societies concerned with the promotion of equality and social justice – given the contemporary global economic and socio-political realities (see, for example, Dent, 2003; Kuhlmann and Saks, 2008). In short, in today's data-heavy, media-saturated, crime-obsessed, risk-adverse and economically interdependent post-recession world, it is important that models of governance appear at all levels (at least on the surface) to promote active and engaged models of citizenship (Wacquant, 2009), not least including digital engagement (Black et al, 2011). The 'accountability drive' that demands that health care occupations justify their actions and that health care systems more effectively risk manage their outcomes, forms just one part of this new political reality (Žižek, 2011). This brings to the foreground the need for academics interested in how the governing arrangements for professional occupations are currently being transformed at international and national levels, to more positively engage with both practitioners and members of the public as they seek to promote a progressive, reforming regulatory agenda.

Tribunal reform, 'the economics of punishment' and the public interest

Recent research into contemporary reforms of the medical tribunal system (see Chamberlain, 2017a, 2017b) has highlighted the need for academics to focus on engaging with as diverse a public audience as possible. In the UK, the GMC is the statutory body responsible for responding to complaints about doctors' fitness to practise. Existing research has highlighted continuing high levels of patient dissatisfaction with the complaint process (Brazier and Ost, 2013). Worryingly, it also seems that more articulate complainants are more likely to get their cases heard (Allen, 2000; Hughes, 2007; CHRE, 2010). Conversely, from the point of view of doctors, research reporting the experiences of nearly eight thousand practitioners found that those who had recently been the subject of a complaint were twice as likely as other doctors to report moderate or severe anxiety, and twice as likely to have thoughts of self-harm (Bourne et al, 2015). Those referred to the GMC had especially high rates of psychological illness – with 26% reporting moderate-to-severe depression and 22% reporting moderate-to-severe anxiety, while 96 doctors have died while facing a fitness-to-practise investigation since 2004 (Horsfall, 2015). Additionally, an emerging body of evidence indicates that pre-hearing investigative measures are traumatising for doctors who suffer from health-related problems. In some instances this is leading them to agree to high-impact sanctions – namely, suspension or erasure from the medical register – before they attend a tribunal, with the hearing subsequently becoming a 'rubber stamping' exercise (Moberly, 2014).

Such findings raise legitimate questions about the nature of the complaint and tribunal process and the impact it is having on both practitioners and patients (Archer, 2014). However, 'the economics of punishment', which is a concept grounded in the white-collar crime literature associated with criminology, offers a useful tool for developing a deeper understanding of the impact of regulatory reforms on both doctors and patients (see Geis, 2006; Whyte, 2009; Hunter, 2015). This stresses that, when it comes to highly skilled occupations that contribute significantly to the national economy and provide essential public services, there is a reluctance on behalf of political and social elites to enact punishment when infractions occur in all but the most severe cases, as the financial consequences of doing so are felt to be too high (Simpson, 2013). For example, Case (2011) found in her study of clinical negligence cases that, due to the severe financial ramifications associated with stopping a trained doctor from practising medicine, in the vast majority of cases a 'redemptive model' of punishment is advocated by employers, medical regulatory elites and the courts. This requires a practitioner to subject themselves to an enhanced level of collegiate and work-based supervision, as well as to complete a rehabilitative skills training programme designed to address any practice-based issues raised. More punitive and therefore more costly measures, such as dismissal and in some cases imprisonment, are reserved for the most publicly sensitive cases. These often draw significant media coverage, such as in the case of Harold Shipman, and serve as a symbolic reminder that justice has been done and the public has been protected from further harm (Quirk, 2013).

Research by Chamberlain (2017b) supports the existence of this redemptive, but nonetheless cost-focused, 'economics of punishment' approach to protecting the public interest. This found that although there has been a significant rise in complaints in the past decade, with the result that more doctors are having informal and formal sanctions placed upon their professional practices by the GMC, there nonetheless has not been a statistically significant rise over time in practitioners being struck off the medical register as a result of tribunal hearings. Furthermore, Chamberlain (2017a) found that, between 2005 and

2015, no doctor was barred from practising medicine for committing serious violent or sex offences, including rape, possession of images of child sexual abuse, manslaughter and domestic violence. Indeed, when action was taken against a doctor for committing a criminal offence, the preferred response was redemptive, with the majority being temporarily suspended for a period of time and/or subject to oversight and monitoring.

The GMC might well feel that in the majority of cases the public interest is best served by supporting a doctor to continue in their employment so they can help to provide society with what undoubtedly is an essential public service. It certainly can be argued that it is essential to allow highly skilled professionals the same opportunity as other members of society to demonstrate publicly that they are 'paying back' society for any criminal misdemeanour they have committed. However, Chamberlain (2017a) also found that the public did not necessarily agree with this line of reasoning. He found that for many individuals the idea of family members being treated by a doctor who had committed a criminal offence was completely unacceptable. Furthermore, in the majority of instances, comparing different levels of seriousness of offence – such as drink driving with sexual offences – did not change their point of view. It appears, therefore, that the public expressed a 'zero tolerance' attitude towards practitioners who had been found guilty of professional misconduct and/or criminal behaviour, and as a result, felt that it was always in the public interest to end their employment in such circumstances. This is understandable given that medical practitioners frequently come into contact with children and vulnerable adults as they go about their day-to-day working life. Nonetheless, it is difficult to conclude that regulatory bodies such as the GMC do not act in the best interest of society at large when they allow a doctor to continue to ply their trade when their fitness to practise is called into question, or even when they commit a criminal offence. This is because, following Freidson (2001) and Stacey (1992, 2000), the primary goal of regulatory arrangements must be to balance the need to both nurture and control professional forms of expertise, and this goal is predicated on the necessity of retaining an element of public trust in regulatory decisions when they are made in good faith. This said, there clearly is a need to ensure that such decisions and the evidence that underpins them is open to public scrutiny (Chamberlain, 2015, 2017a).

It can be concluded that academics should support this process by undertaking a sustained programme of public engagement with the goal of reaffirming the need for members of the public to have more open access to information and statistics about how the professional occupations that provide them with essential public services manage their affairs (Chamberlain, 2017b). At a time of rapid political, economic and societal change, often accompanied by increasing poverty, inequality and injustice, it is vitally important that the social sciences seek to promote greater public understanding of the regulation of occupations that profess to protect them from harm and promote public safety (Wacquant, 2011). This is in part because a degree of mismatch seems to exist in public, professional and academic conceptions and expectations of what is and is not in the public interest, especially when it comes to disciplining doctors when they make mistakes in their personal and/or professional lives. It is against this background, that the chapter now turns to briefly introduce the contributions in this volume.

Chapter overview

The contributors to this volume share a deep concern with the role of the public in the regulation of health care work. Following this opening chapter, in Chapter Two entitled 'Health care governance, user involvement and medical regulation in Europe', Mike Dent sets the scene for much of the discussion in subsequent chapters by examining user involvement in health care regulation across Europe, with particular reference to Denmark, England and Italy. In so doing, he asks if user involvement in health care regulation impacts positively on professional practice and health care outcomes. Exploring the role of 'voice' and 'choice' and the growing role of co-production in supporting user involvement in health care regulation, Dent concludes that the dynamic nature of health care systems and professional regulation means that although user involvement in quality assurance processes has increased, a key challenge that analysts face is ascertaining the true extent of its impact, positive or otherwise.

In Chapter Three, entitled 'The informalisation of professional–patient interactions and the consequences for regulation in the United Kingdom', Patrick Brown and Rubén Flores provide a promising conceptual apparatus, which helps to examine some of the issues Dent discusses. Although this chapter is primarily focused on analysing regulatory and health care developments in the UK, it has broader international relevance. The authors draw on process sociology and reflexively seek to develop an Eliasian approach to understanding the role of public involvement in regulation. In this way, they highlight the value of this approach in tracing the changing nature of public perceptions of self in relationship to the professionals who provide them with public services. According to this view, the 'civilising process' has increasingly required regulators to expand their conception of 'professional skills' beyond the technical and clinical to include 'communicative competence'. Of particular importance is the emphasis this position places on effective practitioner–public communication for ensuring the maintenance of public trust in professional regulation.

Indeed, in Chapter Four entitled 'The regulation of health care in Scandinavia: professionals, the public interest and trust', Karsten Vrangbæk reiterates this position in his exploration of professional regulation in Denmark, Norway and Sweden. In so doing, he notes that proactive public participation in health care regulation is a key feature of Scandinavian countries and appears to be linked to high levels of public trust in professional groups in these countries. However, there does seem to have been an increase of late in the level of public dissatisfaction with the ability of the health care system of each of the countries to cope with the changing and increasingly complex needs of the general population. This is an important point, echoed in the subsequent two chapters, which both deal with recent developments in professional regulation in the UK, albeit from slightly different angles.

The argument that we must not conflate public trust in professional regulation with the level of satisfaction (or otherwise) with the health care service the public receive, can be found running through Chapter Five, entitled 'Medical regulation for the public interest in the United Kingdom'. In this chapter, William Roche adopts a historical perspective on the development of the regulation of the medical profession in the UK, documenting how there has been a gradual movement to greater involvement of the public at all levels of regulatory activity as a result of a series of public scandals. These significantly include failings in care at Mid Staffordshire NHS Foundation Trust where over 1,200 preventable deaths occurred.

In this respect, Roche helps to provide a necessary background to Chapter Six by Judith Allsop and Kathryn Jones, entitled 'Regulating the regulators: the rise of the United Kingdom Professional Standards Authority'. This brings the reader up to date with the state of play in professional regulation in the UK in the wider health and social care context, and underlines how its evolution calls for greater openness and accountability. The chapter documents that this has led to the introduction of a meta-regulator – the Professional Standards Authority – to oversee the activity of professional regulators. In tracing this development, Allsop and Jones highlight that arguments presuming that regulatory arrangements are becoming subject to greater state surveillance and control, with the goal of making these occupations more open and accountable for their actions, are historically and culturally specific.

An example of an alternative regulatory system that reinforces this point is that of Russia, which is covered by Mike Saks in Chapter Seven, entitled 'Regulation and Russian medicine: whither medical professionalisation?'. Intrusive state control of the medicine and health care system has, as Saks outlines, until recently been an omnipresent feature of the day-to-day life of Russia's citizens. Indeed, a perceived close association between the profession and the bourgeoisie intelligentsia under both Lenin and Stalin, meant that it was proactively de-professionalised by the state to ensure that practitioners acted in the service of a communist ideology. Although there have been several moves to reprofessionalise medicine in recent decades, the author details how little in reality has changed in contemporary Russia, and the very real danger that the continued lack of an independent and fully professionalised medical profession may negatively impact on public health in the long run.

In contrast to Russia, in Chapter Eight, entitled 'Patterns of medical oversight and regulation in Canada', Humayun Ahmed, Adalsteinn Brown and Mike Saks discuss how the medical profession in Canada has traditionally enjoyed a significant amount of freedom from state control and hence has had a large degree of autonomy over its regulatory affairs. In reviewing how this has changed over the past two or three decades, with growing calls for the introduction of clearer guidelines and professional standards, the authors highlight some similarities with developments in the UK – including the introduction of formal continuing competency checks by colleges – although the regulatory regime is fragmented between provinces/territories and medical regulatory reform has further to run in the Canadian context.

Regulatory developments in the US are discussed by Ruth Horowitz in Chapter Nine, entitled 'Let the consumer beware: maintenance of licensure and certification in the United States'. In this chapter, Horowitz outlines how the American market-based health insurance system that predominates, with public pressure for reform as a result of a rise in complaints against doctors, is playing a key role in the development of greater periodic recertification of practitioner competence. However, in outlining these developments, she notes the reluctance of state licensing boards to pursue a wholesale approach paralleling that of the UK, which requires all doctors to periodically revalidate their clinical competence. She concludes that this opens up the possibility that the regulatory system might well, in coming decades, become subject to greater federal intervention, although the market-based nature of health care organisation will undoubtedly be a factor in shaping future events.

This contrast in how regulatory developments play out in different countries is also a feature of Chapter Ten, entitled 'Governing complementary and alternative medicine (CAM) in Brazil and Portugal: implications for CAM professionals and the public'. Here, Joana Almeida, Nelson Barros and Pamela Siegel compare the regulation of complementary and alternative medicine in these two countries to highlight how even countries with longstanding economic, political and cultural similarities nonetheless can adopt very different approaches to occupational regulation in health care. Indeed, their detailed and informative examination of how self-regulating practitioners in Brazil define educational standards and practice guidelines contrasts with Portugal where these are imposed by the state. This demonstrates the need for wariness in presuming that the level of state intervention in professional regulation correlates with different types of political system, cultural preferences surrounding health care delivery and/or the presence of neoliberal market-based forces.

Next, in Chapter Eleven, entitled 'Birth of the hydra-headed monster in Australia: a unique antipodean model of health workforce governance', Stephanie Short and Fiona Pacey discuss recent developments in professional regulation in Australia. In so doing, they highlight how, similar to other countries such as Canada, the UK and the US, high-profile health service and regulatory scandals have led to reforms designed to promote public confidence and trust in the governance of professions. However, they also note that Australia possesses a single national system, with a single legislative tool that is operationalised through a unified organisation, which is different from New Zealand, where there is a single legislative tool and multiple profession-specific organisations.

It is left to Jennifer Morris, Jennifer Moore and Marie Bismark in Chapter Twelve, entitled 'Health complaints entities in Australia and New Zealand: serving the public interest?', to specifically compare and contrast these two countries in relation to the handling of complaints. In this respect, the authors accentuate the importance of remaining cautious about presuming that trust is an either/or, zero-sum, game, with one side – either patients or doctors – winning or losing. This is because the public service nature of the work of health and social care professionals means that the effective and fair handling of complaints can increase mutual trust for both parties. Importantly, the authors focus on the role that open justice and data sharing play as the basis for nurturing public trust in regulatory systems.

Finally, in Chapter Thirteen, entitled 'Trust and regulation of health systems: insights from India', Michael Calnan and Sumit Kane echo these sentiments when they detail how a lack of openness, accountability and publicly available information has led to an erosion of public trust in the health care system and professional regulation. This is not least because of the forces of marketisation in relation to medical training and the handling of medical errors. Although they note that the Indian state has increasingly stepped in to ameliorate the situation and more firmly regulate practitioners, they contend that the situation is so severe that academic analysis of the regulatory system requires significant further research before evidence-based solutions can be more fully suggested. In so doing, they conclude the collection of chapters in this volume in the most suitable manner possible – with a reminder that academic 'armchair theorising' must always remain grounded in addressing real-world problems, with all the opportunities for empirical research that they present.

Conclusion

Professional health care regulation in the public interest has undoubtedly become a high-profile topic in the social-scientific study of health policy internationally. It has also been an increasing priority for governments across the globe, in the developed and developing world. As a result, as this introductory chapter has discussed, the following chapters bring an international perspective on their subject matter, covering work from a number of continents, and bringing a social-scientific approach to professional health care regulation, primarily through a contemporary theoretical lens that seeks to build on the traditional 'social closure' model that has tended to dominate the Anglo-American context in particular (see also Saks, 2016). At a time when scandals of professional wrongdoing in the health arena are rife worldwide, this topical volume considers users from the viewpoint of the protection and enhancement of the public interest. Innovative steps to advance this agenda will be needed – ranging from persuasion to sanctions and involving the public and private sectors (Ayers and Braithwaite, 1995). In this and other senses, the book aims to make a longlasting contribution to the study of the professions and the complex relationships between user interests and the wider collective interest in the health care arena.

References

Allen, I. (2000) *The Handling of Complaints by the GMC: A Study of Decision Making and Outcomes*, London: Policy Studies Institute.

Allsop, J. and Saks, M. (eds) (2002) *Regulating the Health Professions*, London: Sage.

Archer, J. (2014) *Understanding the Rise in Fitness to Practise Complaints from the Public*, Plymouth: Plymouth Medical School.

Ayers, I. and Braithwaite, J. (1995) *Responsive Regulation: Transcending the Deregulation Debate*, Oxford: Oxford University Press.

Barry, A., Osborne, T. and Rose, N. (2013) *Foucault and Political Reason*, London: University College London Press.

Beaupert, F., Carney, T., Chiarella, M., Satchell, C., Walton, M., Bennett, B. and Kelly, P. (2014) 'Regulating healthcare complaints: a literature review', *International Journal of Health Care Quality Assurance* 27: 505-18.

Bismark M. R., Martin, A. D., Fletcher, B., Matthew, J., Spittal, A. and Studdert, D. M. (2015) 'A step towards evidence-based regulation of health practitioners', *Australian Health Review* 39: 483-5.

Black, A. D., Car, J., Pagliari, C., Anandan, C., Cresswell, K., Bokun, T., McKinstry, B., Procter, R., Majeed, A. and Sheikh, A. (2011) 'The impact of eHealth on the quality and safety of health care: a systematic overview', *PLOS Medicine*, http://doi.org/10.1371/journal.pmed.1000387

Bourne, T., Wynants, L., Peters, M., van Audenhove, C., Timmerman, D., van Calster, B. and Jalmbrant, M. (2015) 'The impact of complaints procedures on the welfare, health and clinical practice of 7,926 doctors in the United Kingdom: a cross-sectional survey', *BMJ Open Access*, http://bmjopen.bmj.com/content/5/1/e006687.full.pdf+html

Bouwman, R., Bomhoff, M., Robben, P. and Friele, R. (2015) 'Patients' perspectives on the role of their complaints in the regulatory process', *Health Expectations* 18: 1114-26.

Brazier, M. and Ost, S. (2013) *Bioethics, Medicine and Criminal Law III: Medicine and Bioethics in the Theatre of the Criminal Process*, Cambridge: Cambridge University Press.

Case, P. (2011) 'The good, the bad and the dishonest doctor: the General Medical Council and the redemption model of fitness to practise', *Legal Studies* 31: 591-614.

Chadderton, C., Elliott, E., Hacking, N., Shepherd, M. and Williams, G. (2013) 'Health impact assessment in the UK planning system: the possibilities and limits of community engagement', *Health Promotion International* 28: 533-43.

Chamberlain, J. M. (2012) *The Sociology of Medical Regulation: An Introduction*, New York, NY and Amsterdam: Springer.

Chamberlain, J. M. (2015) *Medical Regulation, Fitness to Practice and Medical Revalidation: A Critical Introduction*, Bristol: Policy Press.

Chamberlain, J. M. (2017a) 'Doctoring with conviction: criminal records and the medical profession', *British Journal of Criminology*, https://doi.org/10.1093/bjc/azx016

Chamberlain, J. M. (2017b) 'Malpractice, criminality and medical regulation: reforming the role of the GMC in fitness to practice panels', *Medical Law Review* 25(1): 1–22.

CHRE (Council for Healthcare Regulatory Excellence) (2010) *Fitness to Practise Audit Report: Audit of Health Professional Regulatory Bodies' Initial Decisions*, London: CHRE.

de Vries, H., Sanderson, P., Janta, B., Rabinovich, L., Archontakis, F., Ismail, S., Klautzer, L., Marjanovic, S., Patruni, B., Puri, S. and Tiessen, J. (2009) *International Comparison of Ten Medical Regulatory Systems*, Cambridge: RAND Europe.

Dent, M. (2003) *Remodelling Hospitals and Health Professionals in Europe: Medicine, Nursing and the State*, London: Palgrave.

Freidson, E. (2001) *Professionalism: The Third Logic*, Cambridge: Polity Press.

Geis, G. (ed) (2006) *White-collar Criminal: The Offender in Business and the Professions*, New Brunswick, NJ: Transaction Publishers.

Giarelli, G., Annandale, E. and Ruzza, C. (2014) 'Introduction: the role of civil society in healthcare systems reforms', *Social Science and Medicine* 123: 160–7.

Horsfall, S. (2015) *Doctors Who Commit Suicide Whilst Under GMC Fitness to Practice Investigation: Internal Review*, London: General Medical Council.

Hughes, J. (2007) *An Independent Audit of Decisions in the Investigation Stage of the GMC's Fitness to Practise Process*, London: King's College London.

Hunter, B. (2015) *White-collar Offenders and Desistance from Crime: Future Selves and Constancy of Change*, London: Routledge.

Kuhlmann, E. and Saks, M. (eds) (2008) *Rethinking Professional Governance: International Directions in Healthcare*, Bristol: Policy Press.

McDonald, F. (2012) 'Challenging the regulatory trinity: global trends in health professional regulation', in Short, S. and McDonald, F. (eds) *Health Workforce Governance: Improved Access, Good Regulatory Practice, Safer Patients*, Farnham: Ashgate.

Miotto, R., Wang, F., Wang, S., Jiang, X. and Dudley, J. T. (2017) 'Deep learning for healthcare: review, opportunities and challenges', *Briefings in Bioinformatics* bbx044.

Moberly, T. (2014) 'The GMC is traumatising unwell doctors and may be undermining patient safety', *BMJ Careers* 20: 10–11.

Pan, J., Liu, D. and Ali, S. (2015) 'Patient dissatisfaction in China: what matters?', *Social Science and Medicine* 143: 145–53.

Quirk, H. (2013) 'Sentencing white coat crime: the need for guidance in medical manslaughter cases', *Criminal Law Review* 11: 871–88.

Risso-Gill, I., Legido-Quigley, H., Panteli, D. and McKee, M. (2014) 'Assessing the role of regulatory bodies in managing health professional issues and errors in Europe', *International Journal for Quality in Health Care* 26: 348–57.

Saks, M. (1995) *Professions and the Public Interest: Medical Power, Altruism and Alternative Medicine*, London: Routledge.

Saks, M. (2015) *The Professions, State and the Market: Medicine in Britain, the United States and Russia*, London: Routledge.

Saks, M. (2016) 'Review of theories of professions, organizations and society: neo-Weberianism, neo-institutionalism and eclecticism', *Journal of Professions and Organization* 3(2): 170–87.

Stacey, M. (1992) *Regulating British Medicine*, London: John Wiley & Sons.

Stacey, M. (2000) 'The General Medical Council and professional self-regulation', in Gladstone, D. (ed) *Regulating Doctors*, London: Institute for the Study of Civil Society.

Toth, F. (2015) 'Sovereigns under siege: how the medical profession is changing in Italy', *Social Science and Medicine* 136: 128–34.

Walton-Roberts, M. (2015) 'International migration of health professionals and the marketization and privatization of health education in India: from push–pull to global political economy', *Social Science and Medicine* 124: 374–82.

Whyte, D. (ed) (2009) *Crimes of the Powerful: A Reader*, London: Open University Press.

Žižek, S. (2011) *Living in the End Times*, London and New York, NY: Verso.

TWO

Health care governance, user involvement and medical regulation in Europe

Mike Dent

Introduction

The key question for this chapter is: Does user involvement impact on medical regulation and governance in any significant way? In order to answer this question, it will be necessary to look at developments in user involvement over recent years. Maybe user involvement has meant that patients are being 'empowered', individually and/or collectively, in terms of having a greater say about their health care and where it is delivered than was traditionally the case. This would suggest that user involvement does impact on medical regulation and governance. On the other hand, more cynically, it is possible that users are being manipulated (Arnstein, 1969; Dent and Pahor, 2015) so they feel that they are involved, but in practice their participation is either symbolic or a policy instrument to 'responsibilise' professional autonomy (Fournier, 1999; Dent, 2006a). This means, briefly, to adapt to the requirements of the new managerialism and be demonstrably accountable too.

Before going any further, I need to clarify the main terms used here. Most importantly, 'user involvement' – this I am using as an umbrella term for any form of *active* participation in health care by patients, clients, carers and, indeed, citizens generally (as everybody at some stage in their lives accesses health care services). Moreover, user involvement within health care is a multifaceted phenomenon. First, it can be on an individual or a collective basis (for example, a patient group). Second, the form of involvement can take several forms, some of which includes citizens in general as well as patients, as in the case of Public and Patient Involvement (PPI). And third, the individual and collective approaches can take various forms, depending on whether they are primarily intended to facilitate deliberative, consumerist or collaborative processes. In earlier publications, I have (with others) modelled this terrain in terms of 'voice', 'choice' and 'co-production', and within the model contrasted the potential for 'empowerment' with the risk of 'manipulation' and other forms of disempowerment (Dent et al, 2011; Dent and Pahor, 2015). In this chapter I am revisiting this comparative typology, but with an emphasis on the implications for medical regulation and governance.

User involvement as used here is, clearly, not the same as PPI. This is simply because PPI already has an institutional existence and 'user involvement' remains but a conceptual category, one that encompasses 'voice', 'choice' and 'co-production'. Medical regulation and user involvement might be thought of as disconnected from one another. However, as we see a shift from 'hard' regulation to 'softer' but more encompassing forms of governance, there is increasing evidence that this assumption would be wrong. In their current forms, they are increasingly interrelated. In this chapter I will primarily focus on the user involvement side of the equation and its relations to medical regulation and governance, exploring what Newman (2005) described as:

> ... the focus on ... *social inclusion, democratic renewal, public participation* and a 'modernised' policy process that involved stakeholders from outside government [that] can be viewed as signaling something rather different from both the hierarchical governance of social democracy and the managerial and market based governance of the 1980s and 1990s. (Newman, 2005: 3, emphasis added)

All of this signals a shift from a New Public Management (NPM) model towards New Public Governance (NPG) (see, for instance, Newman, 2005; Osborne, 2006; Ferlie, 2012) discernible within the English National Health Service (NHS). There is evidence of similar developments elsewhere, including within Europe, typically under the rubric of 'network governance' (Osborne, 2011).

This chapter now offers a review of medical regulation and governance before moving on to discuss user involvement in European health care, leading into a discussion of the relationship between the two.

Medical regulation and governance

Medical regulation can take many forms. It was, and to a considerable extent remains, a matter of professional self-regulation and has been core to physicians' professional identity (Allsop and Mulcahy, 1996; Chamberlain, 2017). This was for a long time seen as adequate to reassure the government, citizens and patients, although this has been challenged in more recent times and particularly in the wake of some widely publicised medical scandals. These have included the classic cases in the United Kingdom (UK) of paediatric heart surgery in Bristol (Kennedy, 2001), general practitioner Harold Shipman (Smith, 2004) and, more recently, the poor professionalism and neglect within the Mid Staffordshire NHS Foundation Trust (Chamberlain, 2013; Francis, 2013). Each has played their role in ensuring that professional self-regulation no longer goes unquestioned. Medical scandals are not the monopoly of the UK and all, or most, of the other European countries have required the organised medical profession to introduce new systems of governance in part to ensure properly regulated medical work.

A mix of cost control pressures and the medical scandals already mentioned, has led to an incessant pressure on doctors to extend and reconfigure arrangements for professional regulation to include clinical practice, known as clinical governance (Klein, 2001). The current form started with medical audit (Dent, 2003). This has been developed at least since the 1960s, certainly within the United States (US). Within the UK the move from a voluntary to a formal requirement was the result of a complex mix of forces at work, but became a necessity following the report by Kennedy (2001) on the Bristol case. While the main players were the state and the medical profession, it was the nurses who ensured an audit culture – the first stage on the clinical governance journey that became embedded within the NHS in the 1990s (Dent, 2008). The process starting with the audit culture identified by Power (1997), then became intertwined with NPM and the performance culture that followed in the 1990s. Clinical audit led on to prospective measures of quality assurance and improvement embedded within performance criteria and ultimately clinical guidelines (Dent, 2008) and care pathways (Allen, 2009; Dent and Tutt, 2014). All of this has come to constitute the basis of clinical governance.

Clinical governance, with its focus – in the case of doctors – on the medical work process, is not the only method of professional regulation. The organisation of health professions generally, including medicine, has ostensibly undergone a major change in the UK with the introduction in 2002 of the Commission for Healthcare Regulatory Excellence (Allsop et al, 2004; Dent, 2006b), subsequently transmuted to the Professional Standards Authority for Health and Social Care within the Health and Social Care Act 2012. This ensured that all health professions are now *formally* subordinate to the state and accountable for their performance. In practice, it is the professions, or more accurately elements within them, that principally determine the rules of this new relationship (Dent and Tutt, 2014). Nevertheless, the changes are not simply a charade; they do mean that the members of the medical profession have to accommodate policy pressures on their work more than previously. Throughout, however, there has been the formal recognition of doctors' clinical autonomy, although this is increasingly becoming less individual and more collectively based in the wake of the growing emphasis on monitoring health care quality, initially via medical/clinical audit and more recently with the rising emphasis on care pathways and guidelines (Allen, 2009, 2014; Dent and Tutt, 2014). It is increasingly exercised within a group setting and any individual variation needs to be documented and justified. This system is more one of soft bureaucracy (Courpasson, 2000) than direct control, an extension of the governmentality principle (Dent, 2008), in which the profession and its members retain a great deal of local autonomy but are no longer formally independent of government – a formalised suzerainty.

No longer are doctors able to insist that they are the most appropriate arbiters of what is best for patients, as previously would have been the case. Moreover, user involvement is becoming an essential component of medical and clinical governance. This point should not be overstated, as there is still a way to go yet. One example is the case of medical validation. This has been introduced as a compulsory requirement within several European countries, including the UK. In a World Health Organization *Policy Brief* on lifelong learning and revalidation (Merkur et al, 2008), it is clear that those European countries with health insurance-based systems are the most likely to have established systems of medical revalidation, including Belgium, France, Germany and the Netherlands. Why this is so may relate to the different institutional relations between profession and state within the 'Bismarkian' health care systems, which also relate to pathway dependency. The revalidation process takes place, typically, every five years and is intended to ensure that doctors are up to date with current best practice and generally remain fit to practise (Nath et al, 2014). Within the UK, the process is organised and overseen by the General Medical Council (GMC) and, following initial reluctance, it has now become accepted by the profession. It is largely professionally organised, but does include a distinct element of patient input or involvement. There is some evidence that this is becoming reflected in medical practice – for example, Nath and colleagues (2014: 14) reported evidence of what can be thought of as co-production, quoting one respondent as follows: 'changing attitudes, particularly with younger doctors. So a consultation ... with a patient becomes much more of a dialogue rather than a set of instructions that they issue.'

This shift in doctor–patient relations, it can be asserted, results from the continuing institutionalisation of user and citizen involvement within the NHS in England (while there are similar arrangements elsewhere in the UK there are differences too; see, for example, Peckham et al, 2012). In the next section the focus is specifically on user involvement.

User involvement in Europe

There is now an increasing expectation that the user and/or citizen will play a crucial role in the various processes of governance, particularly, but not only, within the UK. The implications this has for different countries, or health care regimes (Tritter and McCullum, 2006; Tritter, 2009), vary. This means variations in the emerging linkage between user involvement and medical regulation internationally.

User involvement across Europe, for example, has – to a greater or lesser extent – followed a path from *supplication, deliberation* and *quasi-consumerism* to *co-production*. Simply stated, health services have followed a trajectory from a situation where patients are – more or less – powerless, passive recipients of prescribed care (supplication) to one where they are fully engaged as co-producers (and co-creators) of their treatment and care. The established literature does assume that the provision of any service equates to co-production (Brudney and England, 1983) because by definition it involves the user. For example, the doctor will prescribe drugs, but for them to take effect the patient needs to take them appropriately. However, involvement here largely means following instructions and not involvement as is used in this chapter. User involvement, particularly within health care, carries a considerable normative weight; it is a 'very good thing' and often ignores what one group of researchers have referred to as the 'dark side of co-production' (Williams et al, 2016). Arnstein (1969) pointed out that over-optimism around citizen participation often meant that it was only a euphemism or, simply, empty rhetoric. Her view of genuine participation would involve 'the redistribution of power that enables the have–not citizens, presently excluded from the political and economic processes, to be deliberately included in the future' (Arnstein, 1969: 216).

But the redistribution of power argument within the health field is particularly complex and perhaps best understood in terms of the 'capillaries of power' argument by Foucault (1980: 39, 1981: 92-6), which tells us that even the powerless are never wholly without influence. At the same time, we need to be aware of the possible limitations of Foucault's idea of power, with its claim of being productive as well as repressive. Lukes (2005) asserts that this is very exaggerated and 'wildly overstated'. Even so, Foucault's approach is helpful. Latour (2005), following Foucault, suggests – perhaps ironically – that rather than viewing power as 'negative constraint', we can consider it as 'a positive offer of subjectivation'. Indeed, with the theory that Latour is associated, there is good evidence that the outcomes – or effects – of power relations are not always as one might imagine. They relate to the process of 'translation', which has been described as how the matter is 'problematised', whereby people and components are 'enrolled' and then 'mobilised'. Classically, this is demonstrated in the study by Callon (1986) of the scallops of St Brieuc Bay in France.

Types of involvement

Patients, even when submissive, have never been totally quiescent – unlike scallops. Previously, patients were largely enrolled and mobilised primarily in the interests of the medical profession – this being commonly viewed as identical to that of the patients. However, with the rise of NPM – as it became known – within health care systems internationally (Dent, 2003; Pollitt and Bouckaert, 2011), management and governments became actively interested in the mobilisation of users within networks of participation and, ultimately, co-production. This was driven at least as much in the interest of efficiencies as it was in improving the quality of health care. It was also in part intended as a new method of control of the medical profession (Dent, 2006a).

Particularly – but not only – in the Anglo-American world, there continues to be a concern among politicians and policy makers over the general disillusionment with representative democracy and the consequent democratic deficit. Institutional politics has become irrelevant to many people – they no long turn out to vote at elections (Newman, 2001) and at the time of writing we are seeing a renewed voter interest in versions of authoritarian populism. But before we arrived at this point over the past 30 years or more, there have been three main methods of encouraging the active involvement of the public and users in the organisation and delivery of public services, including health care. These are *consumerism, deliberation* and *co-production* (Dent and Pahor, 2015).

The first two reflect key differences between political and market-driven solutions. For the neoliberal advocate, the consumerism of patient choice cuts through the challenges of engaging citizens and patients in meaningful deliberative processes. It is a choice that *appears* to give the patient a meaningful voice, whereas deliberative processes are more indirect, as is the link between the specific patient and the health service. Co-production is an extension of user involvement directly into the work processes of health care, its organisation and delivery. Within the Anglo-American context, 'co-production' (Bovaird et al, 2015) has gained considerable traction, but this appears to be less the case within Continental Europe and Scandinavia – although this may be changing as the Italian and Danish examples that are discussed later in this chapter indicate (Dent and Pahor, 2015). Consequently, user involvement as commonly discussed in the literature is a predominantly Anglo-American and Antipodean phenomenon. It is true that as 'patient choice' it was eagerly taken up across Europe, including in Scandinavia.

By introducing a system of choice, patients could, in principle, choose to go to a hospital that had the shortest waiting list and the best outcomes or simply was the most convenient for them. Again, in principle, to attract patients, and thereby funding, the hospitals needed to make public a range of information around their quality of care, generally for the first time, in order that they could participate. This reflects the Foucauldian 'governing at a distance' effects of the approach, with direct implications for governance.

Italy and Denmark are selected here as both have tax-funded health systems not dissimilar to the NHS system within the UK. The selection provides some insight into the variation within similar systems, rather than contrast with different types of systems, such as the corporate, health insurance-based systems of Continental Europe. To cover the whole of the latter would need more space than available here. Both the Italian and Danish cases are taken from a special issue of the *Journal of Health Organization and Management*, edited by Dent and Pahor (2015). The Italian case draws on an article by Pavolini and Spina (2015) and the case of Denmark draws on the work of Vrangbæk (2015).

Italy

Pavolini and Spina (2015) identify three primary dimensions to user involvement in Italy: hospital choice, user associations and self-help groups. While reflecting similar developments elsewhere in Europe, including the UK, these have country-specific characteristics. In terms of patient choice of hospital, Italy has a much higher rate of patients choosing out-of-region hospitals and/or clinics (in the public or private sector, the latter predominantly comprising not-for-profit religious-based organisations) than elsewhere in Europe. This migratory behaviour is longstanding, dating back at least to the inception of the Italian NHS in 1978 (Pavolini and Spina, 2015), and is mainly a Northern Italy phenomenon, reflecting both historic differences (pathway dependence) and opportunity differences.

User associations are a more recent development and probably provide the greatest voice for patients within the health system. These bodies tend to be disease based (such as for breast cancer or diabetes) and initially grew in influence in the 1990s following the legislative changes enabling the introduction of NPM and the decentralisation of the NHS. These associations were recognised as providing an important element of the user involvement movement that was also part of the new configuration of relations between health care organisations and citizens. In this they contrast to the more geographically based PPI approach in England, currently in the form of Healthwatch (Carter and Martin, 2016). One interesting, and probably concerning, aspect of the user associations is that they are often 'co-created with health professionals' and/or have health professionals as active members (Pavolini and Spina, 2015), which may undermine the independence of these associations, representing more the health professionals' interests than those of the patient. Another concern, not stated in the Pavolini and Spina article, is that the associations may also become conduits for the interests of large pharmaceutical firms ('big pharma') (Colombo et al, 2012), but this is not a concern solely limited to Italy (see, for instance, Rose et al, 2017) although they are a particularly dominant form of user involvement within Italy.

Self-help groups, by contrast, are smaller in membership, but greater in number. These organisations are set up to support predominantly those with chronic illnesses, but also include support groups for patients with rarer diseases. Self-help groups more than doubled in number in the early 2000s (Giarelli and Spina, 2014). Over half have less than one hundred members and are located mainly in Northern Italy, with the largest number in Lombardy. Over 80% operate solely within their region. These are the groups that sit more on the co-production end of the user involvement spectrum, yet the medical profession's response to them is at best mixed, although it may be improving (Pavolini and Spina, 2015).

Denmark

The Danish arrangements for user involvement, on the face of it, are very similar to those within the UK. Yet, while there is progress towards patients playing an active role in the decision making around their care, this appears to be still some distance away (Forde et al, 2016). The main reasons for the gap between aspiration and reality are, however, different from those in the UK, which relate to historical differences (pathway dependencies) in the evolution of the Danish health care system. The most obvious difference is in the specifics of the democratic arrangements that exist in Denmark, which give a real sense of 'citizen voice' in health care matters. These are similar to those found within the other Scandinavian welfare states, but not within the UK. This forms the first of the three governance planks underpinning user involvement in Denmark (Vrangbæk, 2015). These are as follows:

- the historic citizen participation in local and regional democracy (as already mentioned), which actively includes scrutiny of decision making relating to health care arrangements; the more recent innovation of the introduction of patient choice in the wake of the NPM reforms in the 1990s, where the official intent was to make health care providers more responsive to user needs and wants;
- the growing emphasis on patients' rights to information, co-decision and co-management – all of this followed on from the much earlier, but still highly relevant (especially for health professionals), introduction in juridical practice of 'informed consent'.

In Denmark, hospital doctors have retained a certain hegemony in the management of their organisations. That is to say, they have actively engaged in the newer management discourses and training (Kirkpatrick et al, 2009) and adjusted to the new reality without adjusting their work practices extensively. In part this is because the service they provide is already very efficient and effective (such as emergency stroke and cardiac care), but this is not the same across the health services – for example, general practitioner services appear to be underdeveloped, partly because of the disincentives of the payment system. Recent changes being implemented have been experienced as work intensification and have seemingly created a reluctance to engage with patient involvement (Vrangbræk, 2015).

User involvement and medical regulation in Italy and Denmark

There is little evidence of patient involvement relating to medical regulation in Italy or Denmark, in any direct sense. In the case of Italy it is the activism of patient organisations that has come to occupy and dominate this space (de Vries et al, 2009), while in the case of Denmark public involvement in health care is largely via local government (municipal) and regional councils (Tritter, 2009; Vrangbæk, 2015). Moreover, there appears to be little institutional interlinkage between user involvement and medical regulation except in the area of rights to information. More generally, it seems that there has been very little, if any, public and patient encroachment on the terrain of professional regulation. This, it has been suggested, is more due to work pressures than professional resistance (Burau and Vrangbæk, 2008; Vrangbæk, 2015), although this is rarely a convincing argument. Strategies of opposition by the medical profession are often subtle, emphasising common interests, but in the case of patient choice the view was that it was a 'disingenuous' managerialist strategy (Dent, 2006b).

Having provided a basic description of user involvement and a brief account of developments in Italy and Denmark as comparators to the UK NHS system, it is useful to reprise the involvement categories of *consumerism*, *deliberation* and *co-production*, but this time with greater depth.

Consumerism

Seeing patients simultaneously as 'consumers' puts them in an ambiguous liminal point within the health care system. The patient/consumer becomes a 'boundary object' (Allen, 2009) perceived by doctors, citizens, managers and other players in seemingly similar, but often in rather different, ways. Sometimes, for instance, the patient is a collective noun (as a group of patients with the same condition or disease), while at other times the patient is the individual sitting in the doctor's consulting room. Moreover, as a consumer, the patient has choice, but a choice of delimited options dependent on the patient's own willingness and ability to travel to distant clinics. Yet, despite the ambiguity, putting this notion of the 'patient' centre stage effectively rejigs the relations and expectations of all the key actors; citizens have increasingly become 'responsibilised' for their health and wellbeing, including the choices they make regarding referrals and treatment (Mulley et al, 2012). On the other hand, health professionals, including doctors, now have to demonstrate that they deliver health care in a fully accountable way – for example, according to clinical guidelines. This is where clinical governance, an aspect of NPG, plays its formal role in managing the quality of care delivered by the profession.

Deliberation

An alternative to the neoliberal quasi-market solution was the movement for deliberative democracy. This response to the challenges facing welfare states in the 1990s provided a legitimate form of participation that emphasised engagement and transformation rather than a simple aggregation of choices as is the case with representational democracy. It became the way forward for the 'Third Way' (Giddens, 1988) and is seen as a means of transformational change.

The kernel of deliberative democracy is that its decisions are the outcome of dialogue and deliberation (Newman, 2001). The assumption is that the process will be a transformative one as participants adjust and adapt their views and preferences in light of discussion and debate. This would seem to be the hope behind the newer development of PPI within the English NHS. But first the participants have to accept that the forum for debate is not according to party, class or professional interest group loyalty. However, as Mouffe (1999) has argued, this is difficult to bring about and it may be that all one can hope for is an 'agonism of adversaries'. Nevertheless, even where the reality is closer to 'agonism', it is deliberative democracy that has provided the rationale for the forum.

Co-production

In health care, user involvement in its various forms has often been linked to quality improvement, which becomes increasing challenging in the context of finite financial resources and increasing demand – largely the result of an ageing population, rising expectations and the cost of health technologies and drugs. By making patients better informed and more involved in the decisions around their health care, Wanless (2002) estimated savings of around 16% of the UK NHS budget every year by 2022. Mulley and colleagues (2012) commented that this figure was probably over-optimistic, but suggested that if patients were fully informed of the advantages, as opposed to the disadvantages, of intervention then savings of a comparable order could be achieved. From the examples cited – prostate cancer, uterine bleeding, coronary heart disease and back pain – the argument looks to be as much anti-iatrogenic (see Illich, 1977) as for co-production. That is to say, the side effects of medical intervention are more problematic and expensive than managing the disease conservatively. This correlates with policies of encouraging healthier lifestyles, which also inhibit the otherwise escalating costs of health care.

However, all of this is aspirational for, while health care systems are generally struggling to contain costs, none has managed to reduce public expenditure on health (Pavolini et al, 2013). There is some evidence, though, that the average annual growth rate in real terms has reduced (OECD, 2015). This situation is rather different from elsewhere in the public sector where co-production is increasingly viewed as necessary, rather than simply desirable, in order to ensure that services are preserved in some form or other – for instance, by keeping libraries, day care centres and the like open, as well as rural public transport running, and providing a whole range of other services with the aid of unpaid volunteers. To quote the now-classic American paper by Brudney and England (1983: 59): '[G]iven fiscal constraints, citizens are asked to pitch in and help insure the quality of life in their city.'

We can now see this applying to the UK and elsewhere, possibly rationalised as part of the 'Big Society'. Why such social innovations frequently appear to come from the US is an intriguing question. It probably results from the political and socioeconomic diversity to be found across the country, which has given rise to hybridity, heterogeneity and an 'institutional diversity of mixed arrangements' (Williams et al, 2016). This is the country that gave us the idea that there were no 'problems', only 'challenges', and each of the three approaches to user involvement – consumerism, deliberation, and co-production – have emerged as potential solutions.

Each of the three approaches to user involvement takes on a dynamic of its own within the health sector of the country in which it is introduced. There are three distinct and interrelated reasons why this is the case:

- the political settlement that accompanied the creation of the Western welfare states – whether of the 'Bismarkian' or 'Beveridge' (that is, NHS) variety – ensures that health care services have a high political priority (Moran, 2000);
- the reliance on the medical profession for the health care delivered places the profession in a strategically dominant position (Moran, 2000);
- health services within welfare states face unlimited demand with limited resources (Smith et al, 2014).

The conundrum for the state has been how to deliver efficient, affordable and effective health care services sufficiently agreeable to the citizens and acceptable to the medical profession. However, the widespread crisis, or malaise, that has been afflicting welfare states at least since the 1970s brought about a sea change in public sector health service delivery (Esping-Andersen, 1996; Moran, 2001, 2009). Previously, there was an assumption that the doctors spoke for the patients, but with neoliberal developments within the sector, the introduction of quasi-markets and NPM, all this changed. No longer are patients assumed to be passive actors within the system; they have been transformed, at least formally, into active consumers of health care services.

A little counterintuitively, perhaps, given the market principles on which neoliberalism is largely based, one consequence was the emergence of the regulatory state (Clarke and Newman, 1997; Moran, 2001). This was largely because of concerns around the monopoly and power of the NHS and its professionals, epitomised by Le Grand (1997) in terms of 'knights' and 'knaves', where the latter are the actors who game against the system. An example is the case of hospitals finding ways of 'massaging' the official data on their organisational or clinical performance. Within Europe, this evolved initially in the UK under the Thatcher administration of the 1980s (Clarke and Newman, 1997). Sweden and the Netherlands were also early European adopters of variants of NPM (Dent, 2003). Then most other countries across Europe followed suit, with the partial exception of Germany (Dent, 2003; Pollitt and Bouckaert, 2011). It was in the wake of these reforms that user involvement gained real momentum. Early on the patient as 'consumer' became the new focus and rationale for many health service; however, deliberative engagement also played a significant and ongoing role and co-production, certainly within the Anglo–American world, has come to dominate the field of user involvement.

Having presented an account of governance and medical regulation and identified the three distinctive forms of user involvement, the discussion now considers their interconnections and implications.

User involvement, governance and medical regulation

There is a distinctive difference between the Anglo-Saxon 'public interest' and the Continental European and Scandinavian '*Rechtsstaat*' varieties of governance (Pollitt and Bouckaert, 2011; Tritter, 2009), even if this 'bi-polar' is not so clear cut as was previously the case. In other words, 'public interest' and '*Rechsstaat*' are more ideal types than real-life descriptions – indeed many countries of the latter type are moving away from its juridical form. Nevertheless, I would argue that there remains within a *Rechtsstaat*-oriented perspective an assumption that the state is 'a central integrating force within society, and its focal concerns are with the preparation, promulgation and enforcement of laws' (Pollitt and Bouckaert, 2011: 62). This does not mean, however, that the state is necessarily highly centralised, nor authoritarian – we only need to consider the case of contemporary, federal, Germany, or the Scandinavian countries, to see that this is not the case. But what it does mean for PPI – as an example – is that it will be developed and implemented rather more within a legal framework of administrative law than is the case within the UK or North America. Here the law is more in the background and governments, instead, attempt to manage public consent for their policies and resolve conflicts much more pragmatically. This has particular implications for PPI and its role in professional governance.

In the Anglo-American variety of governance, it is crucial for engagement that it be dynamic, even adversarial ('agonistic'). It is, therefore, probably not too surprising that initially the debate around 'user involvement' was driven by a perceived democratic deficit in our traditional model of representative democracy. It was proposed that we find a new legitimacy by developing systems of deliberative democracy (Dryzek, 2000; Newman, 2001). When we compare this with developments in countries with more of a *Reichsstaat* approach, the dynamic has been somewhat different (Dent and Pahor, 2015). However, with the dominant influence of neoliberalism pervading the discourse at the end of the 1990s, deliberative democracy gave way to patient choice as the dominant form of user involvement across much of Europe and Scandinavia.

All of this represents what we can refer to as 'government at a distance', drawing here on actor network theory (Miller and Rose, 2008) rather than direct regulation, and depicts what some have argued, indirectly, is part of NPG (for instance, Newman, 2005; Osborne, 2006; Ferlie, 2012). Not only are these forms of user involvement seen as 'empowering' patients and citizens, they also provide ways of 'disciplining' medical professionals (Dent, 2006a). User involvement provides the basis for the new 'softer' NPG within the sector and it is the language of quality improvement that, in the UK at least, has gained particular traction both in the language of governance and user involvement. Focusing on the English health service, Healthwatch, the biggest official PPI organisation in the country, claims it ensures that the patient is an informed and critical consumer. The word 'critical' would suggest that engagement between Healthwatch and the NHS is more one of 'agonistic pluralism' than of 'deliberative engagement'. In practice, however, Healthwatch is rather less radical than this rhetoric suggests (Carter and Martin, 2016).

It is the link to *quality improvement*, however, that provides particular leverage for users as network actors for it can ensure that user involvement has a direct link to *clinical governance*. This, for instance, could be involvement in the co-design of the care pathways themselves. It is certainly the case that pathways are intended to include points on the trajectory where patients play an active part of the decision-making process (Dent and Tutt, 2014). To date there is little evidence in the literature that this is happening widely. More embedded user involvement arrangements are the patient participation groups that are connected to general practitioner practices (The Patients Association, 2017) and are a component of the governance of these practices – with similar arrangements for other health care organisations. These will be more of the deliberative variety of involvement. Finally, patient choice also impacts on the NPG of health care delivery if it is linked to requirements for good, accurate and reliable information on the quality of care provided.

While I have been able to make the case for the constructive relationship between user involvement and NPG and its components, especially clinical governance, it would be wrong to overemphasise the effectiveness of these relations. With maturity, these assemblages or actor networks may become more embedded and thereby grow in effectiveness. But such networked arrangements always have a degree of fragility about them; they are complex, being comprised of human actors with differing concerns, interests and aspirations.

Conclusion

In this chapter I have discussed user involvement and its relations to medical regulation and governance. The attention has been focused mainly on the English NHS, but within a broader comparative context – in particular, developments in Italy and Denmark.

Voice, choice and co-production developed and evolved in the wake of various, political and financial drivers. 'Voice' in its deliberative – as opposed to the representative, democratic – form resulted from concerns over the democratic deficit in the 1990s, and as discussed in the UK was part of 'Third Way' thinking within New Labour (Giddens, 2000; Newman, 2001). This contrasted with the neoliberals' preference for market-driven solutions, which led to the adoption of the 'choice' model. Within Europe its introduction was initially under the Thatcher regime in the UK, but Sweden soon followed suit, and then choice was taken up across the Nordic countries and much of Europe, shaped by their particular health care regimes (Blank and Burau, 2004; Saltman and Vrangbæk, 2009; Dent and Pahor, 2015). While patient choice has firmly taken root within many, probably most, health systems, it has not been viewed as a complete or sufficient answer to user involvement and the patient voice continues to play a role. Alongside both 'voice' and 'choice' – and 'hybridising' with the former – there has emerged a growing application of 'co-production', particularly, but not solely, within the Anglo-American systems.

The debates around user involvement have been largely focused only on the user and citizen side of the equation. What is less often emphasised are the implications that such systems may have for the medical profession (and the related health professions and managers too). Politicians, for their part, will emphasise what they see as the benefits of user involvement for patients and citizens, but it is also the case that they will also be interested in how such arrangements might be used to 'discipline', that is, exercise some 'soft' control over the work of the profession (Courpasson, 2000; Dent, 2006a). By legitimising patient voice and choice and encouraging co-production within the 'public sector', patients can, and are expected to, influence clinic work and its organisation (see, for example, Coulter and Collins, 2011). This influence, while real, should again not be overemphasised, for it is equally possible that patients may identify more with doctors than management or government – which is an outcome of proto-professionalism in some cases (Dent, 2006b). Even more worrying is the undue influence of large pharmaceutical firms ('big pharma') in the case of patient groups (Pavolini and Spina, 2015). In all cases, user involvement would be counterproductive to governments' attempts to improve efficiencies. More likely is that there will be – and the process has already started – a reconfiguration of health service delivery and a recalibration of professional and managerial control and user influence. If there is a transformation in health care, it could be prompted by leading elements within the user/patient organisations that are the catalyst. But given the complexity of health care systems, the outcome is not easy to predict. One thing that is certain is that medical regulation and governance have changed while user involvement has grown.

References

Allen, D. (2009) 'From boundary object to boundary concept: the practice and politics of care pathway development', *Social Science and Medicine* 69: 354-61.

Allen, D. (2014) 'Lost in translation? "Evidence" and the articulation of institutional logics in integrated care pathways: from positive to negative boundary object?', *Sociology of Health and Illness* 36(6): 807-22.

Allsop, A., Jones, K., Meerabeau, L., Mulcahy, L. and Price, D. (2004) *CHRP Scoping exercise: Final report (January)*, www.gmc-uk.org/crhp_report.pdf_25398882.pdf

Allsop, J. and Mulcahy, L. (1996) *Regulating Medical Work: Formal and Informal Control*, Buckingham: Open University Press.

Arnstein, S. R. (1969) 'A ladder of citizen participation', *Journal of the American Planning Association* 35(4): 216-24, http://lithgow-schmidt.dk/sherry-arnstein/ladder-of-citizen-participation.html

Blank, R. H. and Burau, V. (2004) *Comparative Health Policy*, Basingstoke: Palgrave Macmillan.

Bovaird, T., Van Ryzin, G. G., Loeffler, E. and Parrado, S. (2015) 'Activating citizens to participate in collective co-production of public services', *Journal of Social Policy* 44(1): 1-23.

Brudney, J. L. and England, R. E. (1983) 'Towards a definition of the coproduction concept', *Public Administration Review* 43(1): 59-65.

Burau, V. and Vrangbæk, K. (2008) 'Global markets and national pathways in medical re-regulation', in Kuhlmann, E. and Saks, M. (eds) *Rethinking Professional Governance: International Directions in Healthcare*, Bristol: Policy Press.

Callon, M. (1986) 'Some elements of a sociology of translation domestication of the scallops and the fishermen of St Brieuc Bay', in Law, J. (ed) *Power, Action and Belief: A New Sociology of Knowledge*, London: Routledge & Kegan Paul.

Carter, P. and Martin, G. (2016) 'Challenges facing Healthwatch, a new consumer champion in England', *International Journal of Health Policy Management* 5(x): 1-5.

Chamberlain, J. M. (2013) *The Sociology of Medical Regulation: An Introduction*, London: Springer.

Chamberlain, J. M. (2017) 'Malpractice, criminality and medical regulation: reforming the role of GMC in fitness to practice panels', *Medical Law Journal* 25(1): 1-22.

Clarke, H. and Newman, J. (1997) *The Managerial State*, London: Sage.

Colombo, C., Mosconi, P., Villani, W. and Garattini, S. (2012) 'Patient organizations' funding from pharmaceutical companies: is disclosure clear, complete and accessible to the public? An Italian survey', *PLoS ONE* 7(5): e34974, https://doi.org/10.1371/journal.pone.0034974

Coulter, A. and Collins, P.A. (2011) *Making Shared Decision-Making a Reality: No Decision Without Me*, London: The King's Fund.

Courpasson, D. (2000) 'Management strategies of domination: power in soft bureaucracies', *Organization Studies* 21(1): 141-61.

Dent, M. (2003) *Remodelling Hospitals and Health Professions in Europe: Medicine, Nursing and the State*, Basingstoke: Palgrave Macmillan.

Dent, M. (2006a) 'Disciplining the medical profession: implications of patient choice for medical dominance', *Health Sociology Review* 15(5): 458-68.

Dent, M. (2006b) 'Patient choice and medicine in health care: responsibilisation, governance and proto-professionalization', *Public Management Review* 8(3): 449-62.

Dent, M. (2008) 'Medicine, nursing and changing professional jurisdictions in the UK', in Muzio, D., Ackroyd, S. and Chanlat, J.-F. (eds) *Redirections in the Study of Expert Labour: Established Professions and New Expert Occupations*, Basingstoke: Palgrave Macmillan.

Dent, M., Fallon, C., Wendt, C. Vuori, J., Pahor, M., de Pietro, C. and Silva, S. (2011) 'Medicine and user involvement within European healthcare: a typology of European comparative research', *International Journal of Clinical Practice* 65(12): 1218-20.

Dent, M. and Pahor, J. (2015) 'Patient involvement in Europe – a comparative framework', *Journal of Health Organisation and Management* 29(5): 546-55.

Dent, M. and Tutt, D. (2014) 'Electronic patient information systems and care pathways: the organisational challenges of implementation and integration', *Health Informatics Journal* 20(3): 176-88.

Dryzek, J. S. (2000) *Deliberative Democracy and Beyond: Liberals, Critics, Contestation*, Oxford: Oxford University Press.

Esping-Andersen, G. (1996) 'After the Golden Age? Welfare state dilemmas in a global economy', in Esping-Andersen, G. (ed) *Welfare States in Transition: National Adaptations in Global Economies*, London: Sage.

Ferlie, E. (2012) 'Concluding discussion: paradigms and instruments of public management reform – the question of agency', in Teelken, C., Ferlie, E. and Dent, M. (eds) *Leadership in the Public Sector: Promises and Pitfalls*, London: Routledge.

Forde, I., Nader, C., Socha-Dietrich, K., Oderkirk, J. and Colombo, F. (2016) *Primary Care Review of Denmark*, Paris: OECD

Fournier, V. (1999) 'The appeal of "professionalism" as a disciplinary mechanism', *Sociological Review* 47(2): 280-307.

Foucault, M. (1980) *Power/Knowledge: selected interviews and other writings, 1972-7*, Brighton: Harvester.

Foucault, M. (1981) *The history of sexuality: Volume one – an introduction*, Harmondsworth: Pelican.

Francis, R. (2013) *Report of the Mid Staffordshire NHS Foundation Trust Public Inquiry*, London: The Stationery Office.

Giarelli, G. and Spina, E. (2014) 'Self-help/mutual aid as active citizenship associations: a case-study of the chronically ill in Italy', *Social Science and Medicine* 123: 242-9.

Giddens, A. (1988) *The Third Way: The Renewal of Social Democracy*, Cambridge: Polity Press.

Giddens, A. (2000) *The Third Way and its Critics*, Cambridge: Polity Press.

Illich, I. (1977) *Limits to Medicine: Medical Nemesis: The Expropriation of Health*, Harmondsworth: Penguin Books.

Kennedy, I. (2001) *The Report of the Public Inquiry into Children's Heart Surgery at the Bristol Royal Infirmary 1984-1995: Learning from Bristol*, Cm5207, London: The Stationery Office.

Kirkpatrick, I., Jespersen, P. K., Dent, M. and Neogy, N. (2009) 'Medicine and management in a comparative perspective: the case of Denmark and England', *Sociology of Health and Illness* 31(5): 642-58.

Klein, R. (2001) *The New Politics of the NHS* (4th edition), London: Prentice Hall.

Latour, B. (2005) *Reassembling the Social: An Introduction to Actor-Network-Theory*, Oxford: Oxford University Press.

Le Grand, J. (1997) 'Knights, knaves or pawns? Human behaviour and social policy', *Journal of Social Policy* 26(2): 149–69.

Lukes, S. (2005) *Power: A Radical View* (2nd edition), Basingstoke: Palgrave Macmillan.

Merkur, S., Mladovsky, P., Mossialos, E. and McKee, M. (2008) *Policy Brief: Do Lifelong Learning and Revalidation Ensure Physicians Are Fit to Practise?*, Copenhagen: World Health Organization, www.euro.who.int/__data/assets/pdf_file/0005/75434/E93412.pdf

Miller, P. and Rose, N. (2008) *Governing the Present*, Cambridge: Polity Press.

Moran, M. (2000) 'Understanding the welfare state: the case of health care', *British Journal of Politics and International Relations* 2(2): 135-60.

Moran, M. (2001) 'The rise of the regulatory state in Britain', *Parliamentary Affairs* 54: 19-34.

Moran, M. (2009) 'Review article: crises of the welfare state', *British Journal of Political Science* 18: 397–414.

Mouffe, C. (1999) 'Deliberative democracy or agonistic pluralism', *Social Research* 66(3): 745–58.

Mulley, A., Trimble, C. and Elwyn, G. (2012) *Patients' Preferences Matter: Stop the Silent Misdiagnosis*, London: The King's Fund, https://www.kingsfund.org.uk/sites/files/kf/field/field_publication_file/patients-preferences-matter-may-2012.pdf

Nath, V., Seale, B. and Kaur, M. (2014) *Medical Revalidation: From Compliance to Commitment*, London: The King's Fund, https://www.kingsfund.org.uk/sites/files/kf/field/field_publication_file/medical-validation-vijaya-nath-mar14.pdf

Newman, J. (2001) *Modernising Governance: New Labour, Policy and Society*, London: Sage.

Newman, J. (2005) 'Enter the transformational leader: network governance and the micro-politics of modernization', *Sociology* 39(4): 717–34.

OECD (2015) 'Focus on health spending: OECD health statistics 2015', Available online at: http://www.oecd.org/health/health-systems/Focus-Health-Spending-2015.pdf

Osborne, S. (2006) 'The new public governance?', *Public Management Review* 8(3): 377–87.

Osborne, S. (2011) 'New public governance and public services: a "brave new world" or "new wine in old bottles"?', in Christensen, T. and Laegreid, P. (eds) *The Ashgate Research Companion to New Public Management*, Farnham: Ashgate, pp 417–30.

Pavolini, E., Palier, B. and Guillén, A. M. (2013) 'The health care policy quadrilemma and comparative institutional reforms', in Pavolini, E. and Guillén, A. M. (eds) *Health Care Systems in Europe under Austerity: Institutional Reforms and Performance*, Basingstoke and New York, NY: Palgrave Macmillan.

Pavolini, E. and Spina, E. (2015) 'Users' involvement in the Italian NHS: the role of associations and self-help groups', *Journal of Health Organization and Management* 29(5): 570–81.

Peckham, S., Mays, N., Hughes, D., Sanderson, M., Allen, P., Prior, L., Entwisle, V., Thompson, A. and Davies, H. (2012) 'Devolution and patient choice: policy rhetoric versus experience in practice', *Social Policy and Administration* 46(2): 199–218.

Pollitt, C. and Bouckaert, G. (2011) *Public Management Reform: A Comparative Analysis* (3rd edition), Oxford: Oxford University Press.

Power, M. (1997) *The Audit Society: The Rituals of Verification*, Oxford: Oxford University Press.

Rose, S. L., Highland, J., Karafa, M. T. and Joffe, S. (2017) 'Patient advocacy organizations, industry funding, and conflicts of interest', *JAMA Internal Medicine* 177(3): 344–50.

Saltman, R. B. and Vrangbæk, K. (2009) 'Looking forward: future policy issues', in Magnussen, J., Vrangbæk, K. and Saltman, R. B. (eds) *Nordic Health Care Systems*, Maidenhead: Open University Press.

Smith, J. (2004) *The Shipman Inquiry: Fifth Report: Safeguarding Patients: Lessons from the Past – Proposals for the Future*, Cm 6394, London: The Stationery Office.

Smith, N., Mitton, C., Davidson, A. and Williams, I. (2014) 'A politics of priority setting: ideas, interests and institutions in healthcare resource allocation', *Public Policy and Administration* 29(4): 331–47.

The Patients Association (2017) 'Patient participation groups', https://www.patients-association.org.uk/projects/our-projects/patient-participation-groups/

Tritter, J. (2009) 'Revolution or evolution: the challenges of conceptualizing patient and public involvement in a consumerist world', *Health Expectations* 12: 275–87.

Tritter, J. and McCullum, A. (2006) 'The snakes and ladders of user involvement: moving beyond Arnstein', *Health Policy* 76: 156–68.

Vrangbæk, K. (2015) 'Patient involvement in Danish health care', *Journal of Health Organization and Management* 29(5): 611–24.

Wanless, D. (2002) *Securing our Future Health: Taking a Long-term View: Final Report*, London: Department of Health.

Williams, B. N., Kang, S.-C. and Johnson, J. (2016) '(Co)-contamination as the dark side of co-production: public value failures in co-production processes', *Public Management Review* 18(5): 692–717.

THREE

The informalisation of professional–patient interactions and the consequences for regulation in the United Kingdom

Patrick Brown and Rubén Flores

Introduction

Critical reflections on professional regulation have rarely taken a long-term perspective. In this chapter we draw on insights from process sociology, following in a tradition shaped chiefly by the works of Norbert Elias, in order to make sense of changes in professional–patient interactions and the implications of these changes for societal expectations of health care and the regulation of doctors. We focus this discussion on the regulatory apparatus of medical practice within England, where a shift towards increasing state involvement in regulation has taken place. This widening of 'who regulates' has been accompanied by a broadened understanding of quality clinical practice, with implications for 'what is regulated'. Tensions have become apparent here between the nature of good practice as set out by the regulator and the state, and what is being evaluated in practice by current formats of regulatory assessment. To understand the emergence of these tensions as well as their impact, a longer-term perspective provides especially valuable analytical purchase, as we aim to show in this chapter.

In the section on informalisation and functional democratisation we describe various longer-term tendencies in professional–patient power dynamics – especially the development of more informal, less asymmetric relations and interactions. We then proceed in subsequent sections to consider three key implications and challenges of such informalisation, referring to changes in the practices and regulation of doctors in the United Kingdom (UK) by way of illustration. First, we argue that performances of compassion and care have become more central to understandings of 'quality' practice, as reflected in recent regulatory policies, but suggest that less asymmetric and structured interactions are also less stable – posing problems for quality assurance/ regulation. Second, we consider that while regulators commonly seek to reflect and uphold norms and expectations regarding standards of care, the 'softer' less formalised features of care are harder to capture within the inevitably bureaucratic features of health care regulation and revalidation – for example, whereby professionals are required to show evidence of patient feedback, compliments and complaints. Third, we move on to explore how informalisation processes are also bound up with moves away from a blind, blanket, profession-based trust, underpinned by classic professional regulation, towards a more critical, interaction-won trust. In the final section we consider the implications of new, more negotiated trust dynamics and a wider notion of quality practice for regulating medical professionals amid processes of informalisation. We also reflect on how heightened demands for reflexivity may open up new possibilities for cultivating (professional) virtue through a process of dialogue between social research and health care practice.

Informalisation and functional democratisation

A number of longer-term societal processes have shaped professional– patient power dynamics, leading to the development of more informal, less asymmetric social relations and interactions in the early 21st century. Somewhat surprisingly, such longer-term perspectives have been largely overlooked in analyses of professional regulation within health policy studies and the sociology of professions and professionals. Yet, as we argue later in this chapter, analysing key long-term tendencies is vital to grasping the challenges and possibilities for regulation in the 21st century. Chief among these are processes of 'functional democratisation' (Elias, 2000: 425) and 'informalisation' (Wouters, 2011a, 2011b). Functional democratisation describes the relative reduction in power differentials among different groups and classes as a product of growing interdependence between them. In turn, informalisation refers to a process whereby manners have become 'more lenient, more differentiated and varied for a wider and more differentiated public' (Wouters, 2011b: 2). In the Western world, 'both trends – the decline of power differences and the informalisation of manners – have been dominant from the 1880s onward' (Wouters and Mennell, 2015: 4). As tightly interwoven with and emerging from the processes of civilisation studied by Elias (2000), these long-term tendencies have never been the intentional outcome of any single actor or group and exist amid pressures towards their reversal (Elias, 1996). Yet these processes possess a more or less consistent direction over the longer term (Wouters and Mennell, 2015).

Together, functional democratisation and informalisation have led to stark transformations in how people relate to each other and to their own selves (Wouters, 2011a). In Elias's terms, these processes have changed the social figurations of relationships (socio-genesis) as much as the psychological makeup of individual selves or habitus (psycho-genesis). Functional democratisation has led to a steady reduction (during this period) in power differentials between different groups within and outside nation states: men and women, adults and children, inhabitants of former colonial powers and former colonies, and rulers and the ruled (Elias, 1996). Informalisation has translated into a very different 'emotional regime', a change that can be appreciated if we consider the many differences between the 'peak' of the formalisation process that accompanied the process of civilisation – the Victorian era (Wouters, 2011a) – with today. As an early 20th-century observer commented in relation to children's upbringing, in a statement that is revealing of the feelings of apprehension that older generations have felt when confronted with informalisation ever since the late 19th century:

> The boy of early Victorian days was a ceremonious little creature. He called his parents 'Sir' and 'Madam', and would never have dreamed of starting a conversation at table, and scarcely in joining in it.... One would not wish to see the ceremoniousness of those times revived, but it is possible that we ... err in the opposite direction. (Wouters, 2011a: 151)

In stark contrast to the Victorian habitus of the British upper classes, defined as it was by the metaphor of the 'stiff upper lip', which in turn connected to 'ritualistic manners and a kind of ritualistic self-control – heavily based on a scrupulous conscience, and functioning more or less automatically as a "second nature"' (Wouters, 2011a: 148) – in the course of the 20th century a new type of habitus emerged. Wouters calls this new developing habitus a 'third nature', in order to contrast it with the 'first nature' of biological impulses, and the 'second nature' of controls instilled in the course of the process of civilisation studied by Elias. As Wouters explains, the emergence of a 'third nature' in the process of informalisation has involved (interwoven) shifts in both socio- and psycho-genesis:

The spread of 'third nature' has been embedded in national, continental, and global integration processes, exerting pressure towards increasingly differentiated regimes of manners, and also towards increasingly reflective and flexible regimes of self-regulation. These trends accelerated in the period after the Second World War in processes of global emancipation (including decolonization) and diminishing power differences. Expanding networks of interdependence incited rising levels of mutual identification: ideals of equality and mutual consent spread and gained strength. (Wouters, 2016: 154)

The development of new demands of regulating one's own behaviour and increased flexibility also necessarily involved a new way of managing and expressing emotions: a 'controlled decontrolling' of emotions that 'second nature' had previously taken away from consciousness. As Wouters (2011b: 2) explains, 'informalization also involved rising external social constraints towards such self-restraints as being reflexive, showing presence of mind, considerateness, role-taking, and the ability to tolerate and control conflicts, to compromise'.

What do these processes, and especially informalisation, mean for health care professional interactions with patients, and indeed for professional regulation and virtue, in the 21st century? Put briefly, functional democratisation and informalisation have shifted the power dynamics, interaction norms and thus the expectations of what (good) health care should look and feel like. Processes of reducing asymmetry (Elias, 2000; Wouters, 2016) have led to different demands on self-presentation being placed on both patients and doctors within more informal clinical encounters, with doctors subject to higher levels of informal and formal accountability regarding their ability to meet those demands than was previously the case (Brown et al, 2015).

Part of the new expectations regarding what health care should feel like is that compassion and care have become more central to common understandings of 'quality' practice. Elsewhere, we have argued that functional democratisation can be seen as instrumental in having moved compassion and care centre stage within health policy discussions (Flores and Brown, 2017). Furthermore, in the UK these processes can be seen as implicated in the growth of medical scandals in recent decades (Flores and Brown, 2017). Although the growth in the number of scandals must also be understood in the context of other factors, such as the role of the media and the nature of British political culture, we believe that this rise gives a good indication of how profoundly social expectations of health care have changed in recent decades, and the role played here by informalisation and functional democratisation.

Doctor–patient interactions have become less deferential and asymmetric over time, but also – importantly – less predictable and stable. Brown and colleagues (2015), for example, have shown a generational shift whereby doctors perceive younger patients as less deferential while younger doctors themselves tend to handle interactions with patients in a less formal manner. Combined, these two tendencies render interactions in need of more active negotiation and therefore also more prone to breaking down. While reducing over time, asymmetry nevertheless endures and therefore in various ways it is still the doctor who is ultimately responsible for handling (if not directing) the interaction. The next section examines some of the regulatory and policy implications of these transformations.

The implications of shifting dynamics for regulatory and policy understandings of good clinical practice

The shifts in power and accountability noted in the preceding section can be seen as apparent through, and legitimised within, various UK government health care policy documents and regulatory policies with regard to the effective handling of interactions, as these have come to be seen as increasingly important for quality care more generally. As is most visible in a shift in policy emphasis since 1997 – although also apparent beforehand – UK health policy makers have increasingly emphasised their willingness to regulate health care 'quality' (Scally and Donaldson, 1998). This shift reflects wider tendencies internationally (Allen et al, 2016), with quality usually being understood in several ways (Hansen et al, 2016). One key orientation of an often diffuse understanding of quality is consumerism (DH, 1991, 2003), through which policy makers have explicitly aimed at 'shifting the balance of power' to frontline professionals with the broader aim of enhancing 'the patient experience' (DH, 2001: 1; Newman and Vidler, 2006). A number of policy developments, brought together under the umbrella term of 'clinical governance', were designed with the aim of stimulating and ensuring this and related notions of quality health care through standard setting and performance monitoring (among other New Public Management – NPM – techniques).

While interactions between professionals and patients – in terms of the well-conducted medical interview – have always been critical for quality care and outcomes, interactions as a feature of good health care have received renewed policy attention and intervention. As a landmark policy document captured in 1997: 'Of course, service quality is essentially determined at local level, through the personal interaction between NHS staff and patients' (DH, 1997: para 7.4). Such attentiveness to interactions as a basis of good care is reflected within wider discourses and publications in medicine, whereby '[e]vidence is mounting that effective and empathic communication with the cancer patient and family can influence desirable outcomes in cancer care, which affect patient quality of life, satisfaction with care, and medical outcomes' (Baile and Aaron, 2005: 331). Studies in the UK (for example, Fallowfield et al, 2002) and elsewhere (for instance, Baile and Aaron, 2005) also tend to emphasise the general paucity of communication skills and training among clinicians, and the potential for enhanced communication and interaction approaches to become standard training.

This shift in understandings of 'core' professional competencies has been embraced in the UK by the main regulatory body of medical practice, the General Medical Council (GMC). In the 2002 version of its report on medical education – *Tomorrow's Doctors* (GMC, 2002) – effective communication skills were enshrined as central to doctors' education, as part of a wider move away from knowledge absorption, towards a system of teaching and examining oriented around competencies and outcomes (Brown, J., 2008). So while regulatory bodies have long since aimed to ensure the knowledge and competencies of professionals in the narrow sense of technical-instrumental practices, this has been gradually widened out to include communicative competencies, which Jo Brown (2008) describes as reflecting a change in power dynamics, marketisation, political-policy developments and cultural change.

Not only have clinical communication skills (CCS) become more emphasised within government and regulatory policy, but the nature of that communication has also evolved:

> This shift in society led to the development of a new and more egalitarian relationship between doctor and patient, thus facilitating the emergence of the notion of partnership and shared decision-making. But this change in the traditional relationship called for patient-centred consultations and the expansion of higher order CCS, such as negotiation and shared management planning. (Brown, J., 2008: 273)

Brown goes on to describe these 'higher order' competencies in terms of a requirement to consider a patient's 'illness framework, "patient's agenda", ideas, expectations and feelings' (Brown, J., 2008: 274). Alongside this latter concern with emotions, Smajdor and colleagues (2011: 380) note a similarly growing consideration of empathy, which they critique in relation to the extent that it is commonly seen as an 'essential attribute' for doctors and for medical curricula. These authors go on to cite various GMC advanced training documents, which specify the importance of 'communicating with' or 'demonstrating' empathy in various types of care context (GMC, 2007).

It is in these senses that we see evidence that regulators have sought to ensure that doctors are equipped to handle interactions that are more negotiated and less characterised by deference, following the partial demise of the former 'canons of authority' that had earlier formed the basis of doctors 'managing' interactions (de Swaan, 1981: 376). In line with the theory of informalisation of Wouters (2007), these policies and rules around the education of doctors reflect emotion and empathy for others. Yet there remain a host of important questions about both the appropriateness and possibilities for regulators to intervene around the qualities of such 'emotional labour' (Hochschild, 1979). Regarding appropriateness, Smajdor and colleagues (2011: 380) assert that compassion 'is neither necessary nor sufficient to guarantee good medical or ethical practice'. Drawing on Bradshaw (2009), Smajdor (2013: 116) moreover points to the danger of McDonaldising compassion in attempting to fit this emotion into the 'scientistic' logic that dominates the health care system, a logic for which 'everything which is meaningful must be measurable and controllable'.

Further questions exist regarding the possibilities for training doctors to handle interactions effectively when, amid more informal interactional dynamics, these encounters are less and less within professionals' control. Research points to a growing tendency for interaction dynamics to break down or indeed to develop beyond the control of the professional and to lapse into aggressive patient behaviour and even physical violence (Elston et al, 2002; Brown et al, 2015). So while regulators, alongside and in response to government policy makers and wider cultural tendencies, have broadened the definition of good practice from a narrower instrumental conception to a wider interactional orientation, important questions remain about the possibilities for regulating professionals regarding 'effective' interactions and furthermore regarding the ability of regulators to ensure this.

The implications of shifting dynamics for the regulation of good clinical practice

Not only has the conception of good health care been redefined and expanded to include a stronger emphasis on quality interactions: as the review by Chamberlain (2010) of recent literature makes clear, the very nature of the regulation of UK medicine itself has also shifted significantly. The basic trajectory of regulatory change, which has developed from a rather closed form of 'club governance' (Moran, 2003) to a more stakeholder model (Chamberlain, 2010), has important implications for how we understand the consequences of the shifting notions of care for regulation. As Salter (2007) emphasises, the regulation of British doctors now functions through overlapping systems of clinical governance – imposed by government policy makers – and revalidation policies run by the traditional regulatory body, the GMC. This section develops further the themes raised in the preceding section to consider the limits of an effective 'regulation' of the emotional and interactive dimensions of quality care, first considering the development of revalidation and then latterly considering clinical governance.

Revalidation and a narrow focus on instrumental practice

Alongside changes to the core curriculum for the training of doctors, the GMC introduced a new process of revalidation in 2012, which every doctor registered to practice in the UK is required to undertake every five years. The development of this new format of regulation was lengthy, delayed and defined by reconfigurations of power relations, especially those between the profession and the state (Chamberlain, 2010). As argued by Archer and de Bere (2013: S51), while the 'rhetoric of both parties places the patient at the center of their argument ... the debates that have informed revalidation's history to date have been primarily professional ones about policy, professional governance, and leadership'. Thus, important questions remain about tensions between the use of a language of 'the patient experience' and how revalidation functions in practice.

Early pilot research into the experiences and understandings of revalidation exercises (for example, Webster and McLachlan, 2011) provides some basic though potentially useful insights into beliefs among the various participants. Interestingly, it was the wider features of quality care – 'Improved quality of care; Improved patient trust; Improvement in quality of clinical information; Improvement in patient experience' – which, along with patient safety, were more commonly seen as being positively impacted by revalidation-related exercises (Webster and McLachlan, 2011: 36). What was also evident in these survey data, however, was the stark contrast between very high levels of belief in the positive effects of the new system among the relevant organisations and 'responsible officers' (96% and 84%, respectively, who expected improved quality of care to occur) and the much lower levels of confidence in the new system among the appraisers (36%) and appraisees (the doctors themselves) (43%). These differences could be interpreted in different ways but seemingly those with first-hand experience of appraisals were least positive about their influence and assurance of wider aspects of care.

Annual appraisals are an important basis of the wider portfolio that forms the focus of the revalidation process (Greenhalgh and Wong, 2011). In general practice medicine, these appraisals pre-date the revalidation processes and a recent study by Entwistle and Matthews (2015) of doctors' perspectives on annual appraisals in Wales shines important light on the professional logics through which these appraisals are approached. Drawing on their analysis of text comments within a large survey of general practitioners, Entwistle and Matthews found that 50% of the coded text reflected themes pertaining to a logic of professional commitment to society (altruism and improved practice), while 35% referred to the appraisal in terms of a bureaucratic exercise and 15% reflected a more egocentric orientation.

This latter study does not present specific analysis regarding reflections on the impact of revalidation on patient communication and handling the emotional dynamics of care, but the data excerpts used by these authors do suggest a much narrower focus on technical knowledge (for example, around specific procedures) rather than any mention of how interactions are negotiated with patients (Entwistle and Matthews, 2015). This apparent absence of the more communicative dynamics of patient care can be further understood through the critical analysis of Greenhalgh and Wong (2011) who point to the document-driven basis of revalidation, along with a rather narrow framing of 'medical knowledge'. These authors reflect, in contrast, on a wider Aristotelian conceptualisation of praxis-oriented medical knowledge:

> The 'good doctor' in this context is not someone who collects CPD [continuing professional development] points and meets performance targets (Shipman did this, remember), but a knowledgeable interpreter of situations: someone who takes wise decisions by reflecting on the

here-and-now in relation to a socially shared, historically unfolding, and continually revisited understanding of what, in general, good doctoring is. (Greenhalgh and Wong, 2011: 168; see also Schei, 2006)

This richer understanding of the nature of how doctors 'know' is contrasted with the CPD points model that is integral to appraisal and revalidation procedures, which 'comes dangerously close to being an empty bucket into which facts are placed which produce changed behaviour and therefore patient outcomes' (Greenhalgh and Wong, 2011: 168).

So while the changes in medical education, partly fostered by the GMC, have cast effective communication skills and wider interaction approaches as core skills within the training of UK doctors in the first place, the regulation of continuing quality practice through revalidation emphasises a much narrower, technical and more traditional framing of core medical practice. Central to grasping these policy developments and this inconsistency is one key word – Shipman. Chamberlain (2010) paints a woeful tale of the GMC's slowness and ineffectiveness in responding to warnings about Harold Shipman, a general practitioner working in Greater Manchester, who is known to have killed 215 of his patients. This regulatory disaster has been seen as a fundamental political driver behind the regulatory reforms imposed on the GMC, chiefly following the inquiry by Smith (2004) into Shipman (Greenhalgh and Wong, 2011), which led to revalidation. While poor communication skills can be seen as impacting negatively on the 'private' (personal, non-generalisable) experiences (Habermas, 1971) of health care, they are not perceived as undermining health services or the entire medical establishment. The killing of more than 200 patients, however, was a much more tangible 'public experience' (Habermas, 1971) and therefore was far more influential in shaping policy (see Chamberlain 2010).

Clinical governance: measuring the intangibles?

That the inauguration, as well as the oversight, of ongoing regulation via revalidation has been handled by state and health service actors as well as the GMC and Royal Colleges is evidence of how damaging Shipman and a number of other scandals have been to the traditional institution of self-regulation (Chamberlain, 2010). As noted earlier, Salter (2007) described the significant overlap within professionals' regulation between the GMC and central government policies regarding 'clinical governance'. Recent changes in regulatory policy described earlier have shifted the centre of gravity of medical regulation still further towards the auspices of the state (Greenhalgh and Wong, 2011; Entwistle and Matthews, 2015). Within this increasingly state-centric regulatory regime, clinical governance is arguably more influential in shaping clinical practice than any tool employed by the GMC. We now turn to reflect on the nature of clinical governance and its relative (in)sensitivity to the wider features of medical practice, particularly the handling of interactions.

As with revalidation (see Greenhalgh and Wong, 2011), trends towards clinical governance pre-date the emergence of particular scandals (Brown, 2011) yet the politicisation of the Bristol Royal Infirmary disaster alongside others was a key driver of the timing and format of this policy framework (Alaszewski, 2002). In the third section of the chapter we reflected on the emphasis on, and widening of, notions of quality care within quality frameworks to include interactions dynamics and good communication. Yet given that clinical governance is, like revalidation, also rooted in a particular concern with dysfunctional practice and attempts to identify and correct 'bad apples', we suggest that there is a similar propensity for this framework to neglect the interactive dynamics of medical practice, despite the rhetoric.

In its key aim of weeding out bad practice, as well as in its approach – the setting of standards and targets and the monitoring and auditing of practice in light of these indicators of 'quality' – clinical governance has been likened to the 'audit society' as conceptualised by Power (1997). One salient feature of auditing processes identified by Power is a general difficulty in capturing first-order processes. In place of capturing these frontline practices, second-order indicators are used as proxies in an attempt to reflect medical practice. Power describes how this inevitably leads to various problems of governance due to the varying possibilities, sensitivities and effectiveness of 'capturing' practices on the ground. While second-order phenomena are always compromised in their reflecting of first-order medical work, the more instrumental (outcomes oriented) dimensions of medical practice – as considered through data on surgical complications and misadventures, for example – are arguably less problematic to record, compile and analyse than those reflecting professionals' handling of interactions and communication.

Patrick Brown (2008) has developed such concerns to argue that the rhetoric of the patient experience, while perhaps well intended, is unable to be captured by the rather crude forms of standards and monitoring, and is moreover distracted by the requirements to adhere to standards and to meet targets of wider NPM frameworks in health care. So while policy makers and professionals may both agree that the multidimensional patient experience is vital for quality health care, the nature of the audit system created by clinical governance mechanics creates a quite contrary logic. In place of the more communicative logic of patient-centredness, which many espouse, therefore, a rather instrumental rationality develops amid the 'system' of clinical governance. This latter system is oriented towards the smooth functioning of the abstract-technical and, by its bureaucratic burden and possibilities for unforeseen side-effects, loses sight of features of 'approachability' and familiarity that are so pertinent to experiences of interactions (or 'access points', as outlined by Giddens, 1990) with the profession (Brown, P., 2008). With regard to a wider notion of quality care, 'the government desire for measurement is such an unsatisfactory way of improving public services because what matters is never measurable and what is measurable rarely matters' (Kennedy, 2004: 162).

The longer-term changes in interaction norms that we described in the second section of the chapter, alongside these recent tendencies in clinical governance, which pay lip service to these expectations yet may in practice be distracting professionals from the individuality of the patient, may combine to leave some patients especially vulnerable within recent figurations of UK health care; with disastrous care outcomes emerging as a result.

The most recent major scandal to impact the English NHS took place in Mid Staffordshire, where levels of poor care and neglect led to a public inquiry that came to be understood far less in terms of technical failures and chiefly as a crisis of compassion (Francis, 2013). We have argued elsewhere (Flores and Brown, 2017) that the appalling levels of poor care, especially of older people, which caused such widespread public concern, were nevertheless little worse than more common norms on long-stay geriatric wards in the early years of the NHS (see Robb, 1967; Townsend, 1981; Jefferys, 2000). In this sense, the crisis of compassion apparent within the Mid Staffordshire scandal of the 2010s can be seen to relate to the framing of the inquiry and policy makers, as well as to a significant shift in norms and expectations of care from a half-century earlier. Further processes shaping this crisis included an inevitable lag between shifting norms and institutionalised practices, and the impact of NHS governance and financial management strategies (such as the pursuit of Foundation Trust status at Mid Staffordshire), which in many ways distracted from the patient and adequate staffing (Francis, 2013; Smajdor, 2013). Frail older people – who were found to be especially neglected within the Mid Staffordshire NHS Foundation Trust – may be especially vulnerable amid these multiple contextual factors, not least where informalising interaction norms and understaffing interact to 'require' patients to be assertive in demanding the help and care they need. Stoicism, frailty, understaffing, and professionals distracted by systemic pressures and management demands, may, therefore, combine to create conditions where some older people are left profoundly neglected and harmed.

From profession-based trust towards a more critical, interaction-won trust

In the previous section of the chapter we presented a rather critical account of current regulatory frameworks in UK medicine. We argued that while *prima facie* understandings of good practice have been widened to consider patient communication and the handling of interactions as core features of quality care, this framing of good practice is apparent within changes to medical education and policy rhetoric regarding clinical governance, but much less present within clinical governance, revalidation and related appraisal frameworks in practice. The profoundly bureaucratic nature of these latter regulatory tools renders them ill equipped to capture, ensure and encourage the types of interactive skills and emotional labour that have become increasingly fundamental for good practice (Brown, P., 2008; Greenhalgh and Wong, 2011). Bringing together various arguments we have presented in this chapter so far, we might go further still to suggest that, by recognising and legitimating consumerist tendencies and therefore raising expectations of quality care, these structures of regulation can be seen as combining with wider NHS management and policy tendencies, alongside informalisation, to make care failures more (and not less) likely.

In this section of the chapter, we move to further develop two key analytical themes raised in the previous section, which enable us to shift our analysis towards a more positive and constructive line of analysis. First, we develop critical reflections on the bureaucratic limitations of existing mainstream regulatory governance to consider alternative approaches that may be more subtle and therefore more effective at capturing and ensuring quality care in its wider sense. Second, we then move on to extend the critique by Greenhalgh and Wong (2011) of regulatory framings of practice to further map out what an Aristotelian notion of good practice – as virtue – would look like in professional work and especially regarding the handling of interactions (following Harrits, 2016, among others).

Central to our Eliasian framework, which forms of the basis of this chapter, is the process of functional democratisation and the relationships between interactions and hierarchy as they feed back on one another over time. Eroding, but enduring, hierarchies exist due to the 'inherent asymmetry in the relationship between professionals and citizen-clients, since professionals command a specialized and legitimate formal knowledge and expertise in identifying and solving problems that citizen-clients may have' (Harrits, 2016: 1; see also Schei, 2006). That patients rely on professionals to attain particular solutions to their problems points to a particular relationship between vulnerability, trust and dependence (Brown, 2009; Meyer and Ward, 2013). This can be seen as creating a 'forced option' for the patient to trust (Barbalet, 2009) while this trust moreover places certain moral obligations on professionals (Parsons, 1975; Harrits, 2016). This relationship of hierarchy and mutual obligation – embedded within wider assumptions of expertise, training, professional ethics and regulation – was usually depicted (at some point within the past) as having become rather normalised within many social contexts to the extent that trust was in many cases fairly 'blind' (Calnan and Rowe, 2008).

The reducing power asymmetries sketched in the second section are importantly bound up with a reduced monopoly of knowledge (Abbott, 1988) of professionals whereby processes of disenchantment and familiarisation with medical knowledge are important factors leading to less structured and more negotiated clinical interactions. Informalisation processes, as mentioned earlier, are also bound up with moves away from a blind, blanket, profession-based trust towards a more critical, interaction-won trust. Indeed, while some commentators have referred to a loss of trust in the medical profession, evidence does not so much show a decline in trust as a shift in the nature of trust – from more passive, blind forms of deferential trust to more *active*, *critical* and *negotiated* approaches (Giddens, 1990; Brown, P., 2008; Calnan and Rowe, 2008).

Brown and Calnan (2011) have argued that this reshaping of trust amid civilising processes opens up exciting new possibilities for the regulation and governance of professionals. Whereas shifts in state and self-regulation of medical professionals towards new forms of governance and/or market-oriented models of choice have been legitimised through apparent failings in models of trust (Le Grand, 2003), these policy logics have been based on traditional structures of trust noted earlier. Much evidence indicates the failings of these new forms of public management due to problems of bureaucratic burden, an inability to capture and reflect subtleties of care and related problems of legitimacy (Brown and Calnan, 2011). Yet despite such apparent failings, the possibilities of stepping back to a trust-based, looser basis of self-regulation are generally deemed unconscionable given the scandals that emerged within such a system (Le Grand, 2007).

Yet the reshaping of trust amid late-modernity, where blind-deferential trust has become less common and where negotiated forms of interaction with doctors have become more the norm, makes clear that a reorientation of governance around trust would not be a step back. On the contrary, Brown and Calnan (2011) emphasise the possibilities of harnessing 'conditional trust' as a basis of 'professional obligation'. Whereas prior failings were made possible by a trust that was largely blind and blanketed across the profession, a conditional trust where *individual* professionals are expected to prove themselves to patients and peers alike could lay the basis of new forms of peer-based governance and regulatory solutions.

Organic, self-governed, quality reviewing and improvement approaches, facilitated and resourced by the state but run among local networks of clinicians working in particular specialities (Bridgewater, 2005), would enable a form of self-governing and scrutiny that accurately reflects the nuances of the clinical work, is therefore legitimate, and correspondingly generates far greater buy-in and cultural change (Brown and Calnan, 2011). Within such smaller-scale and peer-led regulatory contexts, paperwork would always be necessary but could be prevented from coming to dominate and define the nature of regulation. This novel regulatory format would make possible an attentiveness to a wider framing of quality, which would not just be espoused rhetorically but could also be accurately reflected in local, less formal and less bureaucracy-dependent peer-review processes. However, more precision and more development are needed around this broader framework of quality practice – including modes of communicating, handling interactions and conducting emotional labour – in order to inform such governance. We now move on to briefly consider some ways in which self-regulation, and wider understanding of quality, could benefit from, and open up new possibilities for, the dialogue between social research, ethics and clinical practice.

Processes of informalisation form an important underpinning for the development of this self-governance framework. As outlined in the second section of the chapter, informalisation has involved the development of a 'third nature', allowing for the 'controlled decontrolling' of emotions (Wouters, 2011a), central for which are reflexivity and empathy. This growing sense of reflexivity opens up new possibilities for social research, ethics and public deliberation to contribute to informing professional self-regulation within health care settings. Indeed, more reflexive health care professionals and patients would be in a better position to profit from tools and insights provided by social research. To give an example, the literature on informalisation could offer health care professionals (and patients) useful thinking tools to better understand and reflect on their social position and the related challenges they face in everyday interactions with patients.

Ethical theory, in turn, could provide health care professionals with further tools to cultivate their reflexivity in a manner that is conducive to the common good. The wider notions of quality referred to earlier, as informed by Aristotelian considerations of 'phronesis' and virtue ethics (Greenhalgh and Wong, 2011), would be one particularly relevant resource in contexts marked by growing demands for reflexivity and self-control among professionals. A framework of professional self-regulation based on virtue ethics would call doctors to (learn to) exercise judgement when, for instance, practising compassion – echoing Aristotle's oft-quoted example of learning to express anger according to the right 'mean condition' (that is, virtue) so as to 'get angry with the people whom one ought to get angry with, on the grounds on which one ought, as one ought' (Aristotle, 2002: 1126b).

In seeking to strike the right balance between too little compassion, which could border on indifference, and too much compassion (see de Zulueta, 2013) – which could, as Smajdor (2013) argues, expose health professionals to compassion fatigue and burnout – health care professionals would need to rely on a practical and pragmatic 'sense of what is appropriate' or 'decency (epieikeia)' (Sachs, 2002). They would need to rely, too, on the related ability to 'know how to secure real benefits effectively' (Hursthouse and Pettigrove, 2016) – in other words, on 'phronesis' or 'practical judgement/wisdom' (Sachs, 2002; Schei, 2006). Indeed, 'phronesis' has been called upon in order to navigate the two logics that Harrits (2016) suggests are increasingly pertinent for many professional fields of practice: a discerning 'logic based on formal knowledge and training, and a personal and relational logic' (Harrits, 2016: 11; see also Greenhalgh and Wong, 2011).

Finally, growing demands for reflexivity in the context of self-regulation tie in well with the idea that opening up spaces of public deliberation about needs and institutional goals related to care can facilitate the creation of more caring institutions (Tronto, 2010). If self-regulation could be grounded on public debate within professional bodies, and with the public at large, this could pave the way for addressing fundamental questions – such as what counts as quality care, what health care institutions stand for, and what needs different individuals and publics have – in a more democratic fashion. As Tronto (2010: 169) argues, '[u]nder these conditions, care becomes contested in many ways, but social provision for care is likely to be better'.

Conclusion

In this chapter we have sought to illustrate the usefulness of Eliasian approaches for debates on health care professional regulation. In particular, we have explored how functional democratisation and informalisation – two interrelated social trends feeding back on one another since the late 19th century – have transformed the character of health care professional–patient interactions, as well as social understandings of what good health care should look like and feel like. In rendering social interactions less structured and reducing power asymmetries between social groups, these processes have led to more negotiated and spontaneous interactions between patients and health care professionals. In more recent years, they have also contributed to bringing heightened demands for compassionate care within health care contexts. Nevertheless, more negotiated and flexible doctor–patient interactions are more open for misunderstandings and potential failures, especially when involving groups less likely or able to demand adequate care, as in the case of frail older people.

We have examined some implications of these trends for professional regulation, highlighting how revalidation and clinical governance mechanisms based largely on instrumental rationality may overlook these growing demands for negotiated interactions and attendant emotional demands, despite the changes to medical education. Alongside these many impediments to the UK medical regulatory apparatus in being able to reflect changing care norms, new and promising forms of self-regulation within the health care professions are also emerging (see, for example, Bridgewater, 2005). We have noted that new forms of regulation may be especially pertinent and necessary where health care contexts are characterised by a reshaping of trust away from blind, blanket, profession-based trust, and towards a more negotiated and interaction-based form of trust. Professional self-regulation could benefit from the heightened levels of reflexivity required by informalisation, its attendant 'third nature' and emerging forms of critical trust (Brown and Calnan, 2011), especially if this reflexivity could draw on insights from social research, ethics and public deliberation. This, in turn, could open up new opportunities for social science and ethics to play a constructive role in enriching deliberation processes related to care and the public good.

References

Abbott, A. (1988) *The System of Professions: An Essay on the Division of Expert Labor*, Chicago, IL: University of Chicago Press.

Alaszewski, A. (2002) 'The impact of the Bristol Royal Infirmary disaster and inquiry on public services in the UK', *Journal of Interprofessional Care* 16(4): 371-8.

Allen, D., Braithwaite, J., Sandall, J. and Waring, J. (eds) (2016) *The Sociology of Healthcare Safety and Quality*, Oxford: Wiley Blackwell.

Archer, J. and de Bere, S. R. (2013) 'The United Kingdom's experience with and future plans for revalidation', *Journal of Continuing Education in the Health Professions* 33(S1): S48-S53.

Aristotle (2002) *Nicomachean Ethics*, Newburyport, MA: Focus Publishing.

Baile, W. and Aaron, J. (2005) 'Patient–physician communication in oncology: past, present and future', *Current Opinion in Oncology* 17(4): 331-5.

Barbalet, J. (2009) 'A characterisation of trust and its consequences', *Theory and Society* 33(4): 367-82.

Bradshaw, A. (2009) 'Measuring nursing care and compassion: the McDonaldised nurse?', *Journal of Medical Ethics* 35: 465-8.

Bridgewater, B. (2005) 'Mortality data in adult cardiac surgery for named surgeons: retrospective examination of prospectively collected data on coronary artery surgery and aortic valve replacement', *British Medical Journal* 330: 506-10.

Brown, J. (2008) 'How clinical communication has become a core part of medical education in the UK', *Medical Education* 42(3): 271-8.

Brown, P. (2008) 'Trusting in the new NHS: instrumental *versus* communicative action', *Sociology of Health and Illness* 30(3): 349-63.

Brown, P. (2009) 'The phenomenology of trust: a Schutzian analysis of the social construction of knowledge by gynae-oncology patients', *Health, Risk and Society* 11(5): 391-407.

Brown, P. (2011) 'The concept of lifeworld as a tool in analysing health-care work: exploring professionals' resistance to governance through subjectivity, norms and experiential knowledge', *Social Theory and Health* 9(2): 147-65.

Brown, P. and Calnan, M. (2011) 'The civilizing process of trust: developing quality mechanisms which are local, professional-led and thus legitimate', *Social Policy and Administration* 45(1): 19-34.

Brown, P., Elston, M.A. and Gabe, J. (2015) 'From patient deference towards negotiated and precarious informality: an Eliasian analysis of English general practitioners' understandings of changing patient relations', *Social Science and Medicine* 146: 164-72.

Calnan, M. and Rowe, R. (2008) *Trust Matters in Health Care*, Basingstoke: Palgrave.

Chamberlain, J.M. (2010) 'Regulating the medical profession: from club governance to stakeholder regulation', *Sociology Compass* 4(12): 1035-42.

de Swaan, A. (1981) 'The politics of agoraphobia', *Theory, Culture and Society* 10(3): 359-85.

DH (Department of Health) (1991) *The Patients' Charter*, London: HMSO.

DH (1997) *The New NHS: Modern, Dependable*, London: HMSO.

DH (2001) *A Commitment to Quality, A Quest for Excellence: A Statement on Behalf of the Government, the Medical Profession and the NHS*, London: DH.

DH (2003) *Building on the Best: Choice, Responsiveness and Equity in the NHS*, London: HMSO.

Elias, N. (1996) *The Germans: Power Struggles and the Development of Habitus in the Nineteenth and Twentieth Centuries*, New York, NY: Columbia University Press.

Elias, N. (2000) *The Civilising Process*, Oxford: Blackwell.

Elston, M. A., Gabe, J., Denney, D., Lee, R. and O'Beirne, M. (2002) 'Violence against doctors: a medical(ised) problem? The case of National Health Service general practitioners', *Sociology of Health and Illness* 24(5): 575-98.

Entwistle, T. and Matthews, E. (2015) 'For society, state and self: juggling the logics of professionalism in general practice appraisal', *Sociology of Health and Illness* 37(8): 1142-56.

Fallowfield, L., Jenkins, V., Farewell, V., Saul, J., Duffy, A. and Eves, R. (2002) 'Efficacy of a Cancer Research UK communication skills training model for oncologists: a randomised controlled trial', *The Lancet* 359(9307): 650-6.

Flores, R. and Brown, P. (2017) 'The changing place of care and compassion within the English NHS: an Eliasean perspective', *Social Theory and Health*, https://doi.org/10.1057/s41285-017-0049-y

Francis, R. (2013) *Report of the Mid Staffordshire NHS Foundation Trust Public Inquiry*, London: The Stationery Office.

GMC (General Medical Council) (2002) *Tomorrow's Doctors*, London: GMC.

GMC (2007) *Advanced Training Skills Module: Urogynaecology*, London: GMC, www.gmc-uk.org/ATSM_Urogynaecology_01. pdf_30452703.pdf

Greenhalgh, T. and Wong, G. (2011) 'Revalidation: a critical perspective', *British Journal of General Practice* 61(584): 166-8.

Habermas, J. (1971) *Toward a Rational Society: Student Protest, Science and Politics*, London: Heinemann.

Hansen, E., Walters, J. and Howes, F. (2016) 'Whole person care, patient-centred care and clinical practice guidelines in general practice', *Health Sociology Review* 25(2): 1-14.

Harrits, G. S. (2016) 'Being professional and being human: professional's sensemaking in the context of close and frequent interactions with citizens', *Professions and Professionalism* 6(2): 1–17.

Hochschild, A. (1979) 'Emotion work, feeling rules, and social structure', *American Journal of Sociology* 85(3): 551-75.

Hursthouse, R. and Pettigrove, G. (2016) 'Virtue ethics', in Zalta, E. N. (ed) *The Stanford Encyclopedia of Philosophy*, https://plato.stanford. edu/archives/win2016/entries/ethics-virtue/

Jefferys, M. (2000) 'Recollections of the pioneers of the geriatric medicine specialty', in Bornat, J., Perks, R., Thompson, P. and Walmsley, J. (eds) *Oral History, Health and Welfare*, London: Routledge.

Kennedy, H. (2004) *Just Law: The Changing Face of Justice – and Why It Matters to Us All*, London: Secker & Warburg.

Le Grand, J. (2003) *Motivation, Agency, and Public Policy: Of Knights and Knaves, Pawns and Queens*, Oxford: Oxford University Press.

Le Grand, J. (2007) *The Other Invisible Hand: Delivering Public Services through Choice and Competition*, Princeton, NJ: Princeton University Press.

Meyer, S. and Ward, P. (2013) 'Differentiating between trust and dependence of patients with coronary heart disease: furthering the sociology of trust', *Health, Risk and Society* 15(3): 279-93.

Moran, M. (2003) *The British Regulatory State: High Modernism and Hyper-Innovation*, Oxford: Oxford University Press.

Newman, J. and Vidler, E. (2006) 'Discriminating customers, responsible patients, empowered users: consumerism and the modernisation of health care', *Journal of Social Policy* 35(2): 193-209.

Parsons, T. (1975) 'The sick role and the role of the physician reconsidered', *Millbank Quarterly* 53(3): 257-78.

Power, M. (1997) *The Audit Society: Rituals of Verification*, Oxford: Oxford University Press.

Robb, B. (1967) *Sans Everything: A Case to Answer*, Edinburgh: Nelson.

Sachs, J. (2002) 'Glossary', in Aristotle *Nicomachean Ethics*, Newburyport, MA: Focus Publishing.

Salter, B. (2007) 'Governing UK medical performance: a struggle for policy dominance', *Health Policy* 82(3): 263-75.

Scally, G. and Donaldson, L. J. (1998) 'Clinical governance and the drive for quality in the new NHS in England', *British Medical Journal* 317: 61-5.

Schei, E. (2006) 'Doctoring as leadership: the power to heal', *Perspectives in Biology and Medicine* 49(3): 393-406.

Smajdor, A. (2013) 'Reification and compassion in medicine: a tale of two systems', *Clinical Ethics* 8(4): 111-18.

Smajdor, A., Stöckl, A. and Salter, C. (2011) 'The limits of empathy: problems in medical education and practice', *Journal of Medical Ethics* 37(6): 380-3.

Smith, J. (2004) *The Shipman Inquiry: Fifth Report: Safeguarding Patients: Lessons from the Past – Proposals for the Future*, Cm 6394, London: The Stationery Office.

Townsend, P. (1981) 'The structured dependency of the elderly: a creation of social policy in the twentieth century', *Ageing and Society* 1(1): 5-28.

Tronto, J. C. (2010) 'Creating caring institutions: politics, plurality, and purpose', *Ethics and Social Welfare* 4(2): 158-71.

Webster, M. and McLachlan, J. (2011) *Independent Evaluation of the Medical Revalidation Pathfinder Pilot: Final Report*, London: Department of Health.

Wouters, C. (2007) *Informalization: Manners and Emotions since 1980*, London: Sage.

Wouters, C. (2011a) 'How civilizing processes continued: towards an informalization of manners and a third nature personality', *Sociological Review* 59(1): 140-59.

Wouters, C. (2011b) 'Informalisation', in Southerton, D. (ed) *Encyclopedia of Consumer Culture*, London: Sage.

Wouters, C. (2016) 'Functional democratisation and disintegration as side-effects of differentiation and integration processes', *Human Figurations* 5(2), http://hdl.handle.net/2027/spo.11217607.0005.208

Wouters, C. and Mennell, S. (2015) 'Discussing theories and processes of civilisation and informalisation: criteriology', *Human Figurations* 4(3), http://hdl.handle.net/2027/spo.11217607.0004.302

The regulation of health care in Scandinavia: professionals, the public interest and trust

Karsten Vrangbæk

Introduction

The three Scandinavian countries – Denmark, Norway and Sweden – are characterised by extensive welfare services, cultural similarities and close historical links. The countries also share a continued commitment to public involvement in the financing and delivery of health care. The aim is to support key values of universalism and equal access. Due to the reliance on public financing and universalist ideas, the governance structure is based on democratic decision making at state, regional and municipal levels. The Scandinavian countries are often portrayed as having a high general level of trust within the population, and between citizens and the state. This is often ascribed to a low level of corruption in the public sector and the high level of homogeneity in the population (Rothstein, 2011).

The institutional structure of health care in the three Scandinavian states is important for understanding the regulation of health professionals and the relationship between them and the public. Given the high degree of public involvement and the generally high levels of trust in the public sector, one might expect that conditions for serving the public interest are particularly good in the Scandinavian health systems. Similarly, one might expect that public involvement in regulating and providing health care facilitates a high level of trust between patients and health professionals, as there is little direct economic interaction between the two groups. The aim of this chapter is to explore the evidence about such claims and discuss the reasons behind the results. To facilitate the analysis, we start out by describing key features of the institutional structure of Scandinavian health care systems and the regulation of health professionals.

The institutional structure of Scandinavian health care systems

As Vrangbæk (2017) has noted in terms of the institutional structure of Scandinavian health care systems, traditionally the political culture of such countries has been based on a broad consensus behind the welfare state idea. Consequently, the health systems are based on the principles of universality and equity. All inhabitants have equal rights to public health services, whatever their social status or geographic location. This persistent emphasis on equity has been combined with a tradition of democratic management at the decentralised level, with a key role for regions and municipalities in delivering health care. Regions own and operate almost all of the hospitals in the three countries. Municipalities provide a broad range of welfare services, including social care, elder care, long-term care and various prevention, rehabilitation and health promotion activities. General practitioners (GPs) are private enterprises in Denmark and Norway, but operate within a public governance framework and general agreements with the regional authorities. Sweden has a slightly different model based on a combination of public health centres and private enterprises for the delivery of primary care.

Scandinavian health care systems are tax-funded with no risk- or premium-based financing. This is because there is only a minor connection between individual health risks and costs, which are limited to out-of-pocket payments, with voluntary health insurance traditionally playing a limited role, except as coverage for co-payments or to pay for services that are not fully covered by the public system. Around 40% of all Danes have purchased complementary insurance, mostly to cover co-payments. A potentially more important development is the rapid increase in supplementary/duplicate voluntary health insurance (VHI), which provides fast access to private diagnostic and treatment services. Around 20% of all citizens in Denmark are covered by this type of insurance. The corresponding figures are 9% in Norway and 7% in Sweden (Alexandersen et al, 2016).

In spite of the growth in VHI, there is still rather limited use of private health care services. Unlike in many other European countries, there is no strong tradition for private not-for-profit hospitals, and only a handful of those exist (Øvretveit, 2003). Private for-profit clinics and hospitals have grown in numbers in the past two decades, but still only represent a fraction (less than 5%) of total capacity, although some medical specialties have more private involvement than others.

Patients' rights have been important in the health care policy debate in Scandinavia, and all three countries have extensive legislation on patients' rights. Another common feature is the introduction of patient choice of hospital. This was introduced in all three countries during the 1990s. In addition, all three countries have introduced waiting time (or treatment) guarantees to address persistent issues of long waiting times. The Danish diagnosis guarantee provides access to foreign or private treatment facilities if the expected waiting time at public hospitals exceeds one month (less for life-threatening diseases).

Governance and formal responsibility for the provision of health services

The governance of Scandinavian health care systems takes place in a multi-level structure involving national authorities, regions and municipalities (see Table 4.1). The national level is in charge of the legislative framework and has an important role in coordinating the development of guidelines and general policies. There are institutionalised forums for negotiation between decentralised authorities and the state in all three countries. These negotiations are tied to the budgeting agreements between the state and the associations for regions and municipalities. The economic steering power of the state has been strengthened over the past decade through formal legislation and tighter control over the allocation of funding – particularly in Denmark and Norway, where the regions no longer have the ability to issue taxes. The counties in Sweden have a relatively larger degree of autonomy, which has resulted in different organisational and managerial models across the country. This is important in relation to the issue of the public interest, where Denmark and Norway have gradually shifted to a strategy of more centralised control as a way to pursue the public interest, while Sweden so far has maintained the official position – that county-level differentiation according to local political preferences is the best way to do this.

The reforms in Denmark and Norway have introduced significant differences in the health care structures of the respective countries, reflecting the constant evolution of the Scandinavian models through incremental and more radical change processes (Magnussen et al, 2009). One quite striking difference is related to the number and size of regions and municipalities. In 2007, Denmark underwent a comprehensive public sector reform that moved responsibility for hospital and primary care services from the counties to five new and larger regions and reduced the number of municipalities from 271 to 98, most of them

Table 4.1: Governance and formal responsibilities

	Denmark	**Sweden**	**Norway**
Formal legislative frame	State	State	State
Surveillance, guidelines and general performance targets	State; negotiated agreements between state and regions	State	State; negotiated contracts with regional health enterprises
Hospital care	Regions (5) with democratically elected boards	Counties (18) with democratically elected councils	Health regions (4) with state appointed boards
Primary care	Regions: General agreements with privately owned general and specialist practices	Counties: Public health centers and salaried general practitioners	Municipalities: General agreements with privately owned general and specialist practices
Public health: Prevention and health promotion. Rehabilitation outside hospitals	State and municipalities	State and municipalities	State and municipalities

Source: Own compilation based on European Observatory on Health Systems HiT reports for Denmark, Sweden and Norway (http://www.euro.who.int/en/about-us/partners/observatory/publications/health-system-reviews-hits)

with more than 30,000 inhabitants. The idea was to achieve benefits of scale and to create municipal units of sufficient size to finance and provide a broad range of home care, rehabilitation and long-term care services, allowing the regions to optimise hospital services by reducing in-hospital admission time and convert more services to ambulatory care. A Norwegian reform in 2002 created five (now four) regions, but maintained a high number of municipalities of very different sizes. Sweden is considering a similar type of structural reform to create regions instead of the current counties.

All three countries are restructuring their hospital infrastructure through amalgamations, reorganisation and the building of new hospitals. In Denmark, the hospital structure has been reorganised since 2007, resulting in fewer and larger hospitals (from 82 geographical locations in 2007 to 68 in 2016, some of which are joined into the same hospital organisation). The number of acute hospitals has been reduced from about 40–45 to 21 (Christiansen and Vrangbæk, 2018, under review). At the same time, a major government investment scheme has been launched. New hospitals are currently under construction in all five Danish regions in addition to comprehensive projects to renew or enlarge existing hospitals. This development is interesting, as it represents a shift in thinking about public interests. Previously there was a strong emphasis on proximity and local management, guided by regional democratic processes. The centralisation trend represents a stronger belief in benefits of scale and centralisation as a way to pursue the public interest, which tends to be perceived in output terms rather than process dimensions.

The structural reforms and the centralisation of hospital infrastructure have been spurred by several factors. Most important has been the increasing financial burden placed on governments as a result of increasing demand pressure, expensive new medical technology and ageing populations. Other factors include the need to deal with growing numbers of chronic care patients by enhancing the care capacity in the municipalities and a desire to improve coordination between health care and other welfare services such as social care.

Financing and payment schemes

All three countries predominantly rely on public financing of health services. Because of adherence to the overall principles of equity and universal coverage, there is limited user payment. In Denmark, this is mostly concentrated on pharmaceuticals and dental services, while both Norway and Sweden have a nominal fee for consultations in primary care and admissions to hospital. National taxation is the primary source of funding in Denmark and Norway, whereas Sweden is more decentralised in terms of financing. National funding is redistributed to decentralised authorities in the form of block grants calculated on 'objective criteria', such as population size and composition and activity-based funding. Norway has been most willing to experiment with activity-based financing for hospitals.

Payments to GPs in Norway and Denmark are based on nationally negotiated tariffs that determine the fees for different services. In Denmark, they are paid a combination of fee for service (about two thirds of their income) and capitation payment. The bi-annual negotiations between the association for general practitioners and the association of regions include agreements on such items as policy initiatives, the regulation of quality and data sharing. In this sense, the negotiations and agreements are important general policy arenas for developing the regulation of health professionals, and for balancing state, professional and patient interests.

The regulation of professionals

Most hospital doctors in Scandinavia are employed as salaried personnel in public hospitals. Employment contracts for health professionals specify duties and rights, while their public employers have the right to organise and manage the work. Public managers are also responsible for hiring and firing hospital staff. This relationship means that public authorities have direct access to influence professional practices through their status as employers. The bureaucratic structures of regions and hospitals are thus the primary mode of the regulation of health professionals in hospitals. This type of regulation focuses on operational issues as well as economic, productivity and quality dimensions of health care.

In addition to the employment–based management of professionals there is external public regulation of professionals and health care organisations. This regulation is organised as external oversight by national–level authorities that are responsible for the licensing of health professionals, and for intervening in the case of malpractice or quality breaches in health care organisations and by individual health care professionals. National authorities can issue warnings and ultimately revoke the licences to practice for individual health care professionals.

Clinical performance data, patient experience data and activity data are used to support administrative and political accountability at several levels. Hospital management provides internal accountability forums in hospital organisations, while regional/county and national authorities are forums for holding hospital departments and hospital managers to account. In this sense, we can observe a chain of accountability structures, where lower–level forums become accountable to forums at higher levels, and where performance measurements are important in the process of debate and potential interventions. Some interventions, particularly in regards to (economic) activity performance are 'automatic', while others are ad–hoc adjustments based on strategic deliberations or performance measurement data.

Accountability relations also include external stakeholders, the media and the population at large. This is sometimes labelled 'political accountability' and sometimes 'public accountability' (Bovens, 2007). Performance measures are posted on the internet, and published in benchmarking reports by public authorities in order to facilitate comparison and choice. The 'forums' in this case include organisations, the media and individuals, and debate on the results may be more or less structured.

Performance measurements have thus become an integrated part of the system, and have strengthened the knowledge base for the regulation of professionals. Yet, it is also clear that the different uses of performance data for internal development and external accountability can create tensions within the organisations. Individuals and organisations are much more likely to engage in strategic reporting practices, or react by 'goal displacement' and 'tunnel vision', if they know that measures may result in sanctions or rewards (Bevan and Hood, 2009).

The overlap of internal and external regulation structures is particularly relevant at the hospital management and regional administration levels (Klenk et al, 2016). Hospital management must balance resources and attention devoted to the different accountability relations at different times, and they must implement internal management systems to encourage health professionals to deliver data to the various systems. This is not trivial as many health professionals question the benefit of the many reporting requirements compared with the costs in terms of time consumption. In essence, they argue that the transaction and administrative costs are too high, and that it 'takes time away from patient contact and core activities' (Obel and Lintz, 2012, np). However, the medical association and the national elites have tended to support quality assessment schemes, although they also emphasise that the effort must match the expected benefits, and that the burdens should not be overly onerous for individual doctors.

In recognition of the growing critique from health professionals, there was a significant change in the regulatory set-up for quality management in Denmark in 2016. The accreditation-based scheme involved periodic assessments according to a significant number of nationally developed standards. However, health professionals complained that the standards were too inflexible and too far removed from their understanding of quality. Furthermore, they pointed to the significant amount of resources being spent on documentation and inspection. The government decided to accommodate the critique. The result was an agreement to abandon the accreditation-based scheme, and replace this with a scheme consisting of fewer national targets, combined with locally determined performance regulation schemes. Meanwhile, all regions are experimenting with various types of 'value-based payment' schemes for hospitals, partly inspired by the ideas of Michael Porter, an influential American professor of Management and Economics at Harvard Business School. His ideas about value based health care are widely referenced throughout the world. The new local quality regulation schemes are supposed to feed into these new incentive structures.

Patient involvement in the regulation of health organisations and professionals

Patient involvement in the Scandinavian health system is based on the mechanisms of choice, voice and co-production (Dent et al, 2011; Vrangbæk, 2015). These will now be considered in turn.

Choice

Choice of public hospital upon referral was introduced in 1993. This was partly a response to international trends of marketisation, and partly a pragmatic way of dealing with growing dissatisfaction with long waiting times in some facilities (Vrangbæk, 1999). Concerns about waiting times exceeding political expectations led to the introduction of a waiting time guarantee in 2002. In its current version, this entails publicly funded treatment at private hospitals/clinics, if the public system is unable to provide a diagnosis (or a plan for diagnosis) within one month, and subsequent treatment within one month. The choice of hospitals is supported by e-health portals with service and quality information (esundhed.dk). This portal also allows a tailored comparison of hospitals in terms of waiting times and selected quality dimensions.

Voice

Patients can voice their opinions as citizens and voters through the ordinary democratic channels at municipal, regional (county) and state levels and via direct interaction with health care organisations and professionals. The three Scandinavian countries have been at the forefront of establishing formal rights for citizens in their relationship to the health system. Using Denmark as a case study country, we can observe several general mechanisms for patient involvement. First, patients have a number of opportunities for impact through voice mechanisms. The right to access personal health records is written into national Danish health law. Hospitals are also obliged to inform patients about treatment options and risks, and to collect informed consent, before treatment. The rules about informed consent were introduced into Danish judicial practice in the 1970s and codified into law in 1992 (Jacobsen et al, 2008). It is further specified that information must be provided on an ongoing basis and that it must be in a format that is comprehensible for the patient (Pedersen and Kirk, 2014). Such formal rules about informed consent have become part of a broader model for shared decision making, which can also be found in Australia, Canada, England, Germany and the Netherlands. This particular articulation of patient involvement can thus also be seen as an example of the international diffusion of a 'fashionable idea' within health care (Røvik, 1998; Sahlin and Wedlin, 2008).

A follow-up to the general principle of informed consent is the more ambitious idea of developing truly 'shared decision making' in all interactions between health professionals and patients. The 'shared decision model' implies that health professionals must inform patients about medical options and risks and invite them to participate in the weighing of treatment alternatives to suit individual preferences. Individual patient perspectives, preferences and rights must be taken into consideration in this dialogue between patients and health professionals. The idea is to facilitate a 'partnership' between the patient and the health professional, whereby the best treatment pathway is selected for the individual patient (Jacobsen et al, 2008). The fact that this idea has penetrated so quickly into national policy circles probably indicates that, in spite of the early emphasis on patient involvement in Denmark, there are considerable shortcomings in the practical implementation of an informed dialogue between health care professionals and patients. In this sense, the power and knowledge asymmetry appears to be an enduring barrier. In principle, the ideas and practices of shared decision-making provide very good opportunities for patient involvement in managing health, yet there are indications that they are easier to use for some patients than others (Martin, 2010), and that implementation of the joint decision model varies considerably across the country (Jacobsen et al, 2008).

Scandinavians also have the right to voice their opinions through democratic processes and elections to national, regional and local-level democratic assemblies. The regional and local councils are particularly relevant for health care issues, and voting participation remains relatively high. The decentralised democracy means that it is relatively easy to approach elected officials, although distances have become larger with the Danish and Norwegian reforms, which have led to diminishing confidence in being able to influence decisions, at least in the Danish case (Hjelmar and Hansen, 2013). Many patients are members of patient organisations and other non-governmental organisations that aggregate patient voices to influence politicians and parties. Patient organisations typically perform the dual roles of providing information and service to their members and working as interest organisations to influence policy making. Patient organisations participate in many committees and councils in the corporatised structure (Opedal et al, 2012).

It is also quite common for regions and hospitals to work with more deliberative forums for participation from patients and citizens. Norwegian hospitals have user representatives on their boards, and Danish regions have developed concepts of citizen forums and direct lines to management. Another type of direct possibility for voicing opinions is through the patient satisfaction surveys that are conducted at regular intervals by regions and hospitals. These surveys are used in the ongoing dialogue about service development. A more direct type of patient involvement in the regulation of health professionals is via the formal complaint system. In all of the Scandinavian countries, complaints are mainly handled within the public sector and only rarely involve referral to the civic court system. Taking the Danish case as an example, there are three different elements in handling a patient complaint. First, the patient must decide whether the complaint involves a treatment facility or a health care professional. Initially, a decision is made by administrative staff at the national level. Decisions are then made as appropriate in a further stage in a council with the representation of patients and professionals. In both cases the decisions are made public and are also referred to the relevant (regional, municipal or state) authority for further action. The issue of compensation is another element in the evaluation of complaints. This is dealt with by a separate national authority, supported by independent professional experts.

Co-production

The 'co-production' of health services has emerged as a much-praised, but often disappointing innovation in the practice of health care (Jacobsen et al, 2008; Dunston et al, 2009). The core of the concept is the active involvement of citizens (patients) in producing public services together with public organisations (Pestoff, 2012). Arguably, some level of co-production has always been part of health care delivery. Rehabilitation necessarily involves the active involvement of patients. Diagnosing and treating patients has always required some degree of interactive dialogue. Yet the combination of demographic and epidemiological changes with growing numbers of citizens with chronic care needs, resource constraints and new technology has led to a growing interest in other new types of co-production. These often involve e-health and telecare solutions with home-based monitoring and e-based communication between patients and health professionals. This is particularly relevant for chronic care patients and citizens in old age, where digital solutions can be used for ongoing monitoring and adjustment to prevent deterioration and manage the patient's disease. Examples include home-based monitoring devices for chronic obstructive pulmonary disease, diabetes including diabetic ulcers, and heart diseases (Vrangbæk, 2015).

Does regulation promote the public interest in Scandinavia?

A key dilemma in public health care systems is that the public interest is a relatively ambiguous concept that can be interpreted differently according to different underlying value orientations. Most people would probably agree that high-quality services for the individual and improved population health are among the core objectives of health systems. Any activity that increases these parameters would therefore support the public interest. However, many citizens would also agree that it is important that these goals are pursued in the most efficient manner. Taking resource consumption into consideration serves a particular view of the public interest, and speaks to the interests of taxpayers. Yet, from a health professional perspective, such considerations may lead to undue restrictions on access or the availability of technology and thus be counterproductive in the pursuit of the public interest. Some citizens would also emphasise equity as a core public interest. This is based on ideas of moral obligations to take care of all citizens, regardless of their ability to pay, or their value to society. Others would emphasise individuality and the right to choose the service level that suits individual preferences. From this perspective, health care should be seen in terms of a market and competition, and it is believed that choice and competition will be the most effective way to serve the public interest.

These examples illustrate that the public interest is a contested concept, and that the different interpretations can have very different implications for the organisation of health care. The dualistic regulatory structure described in the previous sections aims to balance different underlying objectives and perceptions of the public interest in Scandinavian health care systems. The hierarchical management structure, with its emphasis on democratic management and public service hierarchies, aims to promote the public interest as citizens can influence politicians in their collective decision making. Politicians are responsible for managing the health systems through the public bureaucracies. Health professionals in hospitals and municipalities are employed within public hierarchies and are thus part of this chain of command. Hospital managers, bureaucratic managers and ultimately politicians are supposed to intervene if health professionals or organisations fail to live up to their obligations according to the public interest. In this sense, the Scandinavian health systems have rather strong provisions for securing the public interest

Individual patient quality and protection against professional misconduct lie within the profession-oriented regulation system, with the national health authorities at the highest level, and typically with a network of regionally based health officers as described earlier. The national authorities have historically been staffed by health professionals, and they collaborate with medical societies and experts when developing guidelines and indicators for the assessment of quality. In this sense, there is a long tradition of the integration of health professionals in the public bureaucracy. However, recent years have seen an increasing number of administrative staff (such as political scientists and lawyers) and numerous reorganisations of the national health authorities, particularly in Denmark and Norway. This has created tensions and debates and has contributed to a gradual rebalancing of the professional and the general public administration interests in the system.

All in all, it appears that the conditions for pursuing the public interest are quite good due to the democratic and public management structures, and the emphasis on transparency in decision making. However, there are also ongoing battles about definitions of the public good as seen from the perspectives of different patient groups, health professionals, bureaucrats and politicians. The democratic system provides a structure for weighing such perspectives against each other.

Does the system provide a high level of trust between patients and health professionals?

Trust is a multidimensional phenomenon, which can only be measured indirectly. At its core, it is a dualistic relationship between a patient and a health professional, which is highly dependent on individual expectations, previous experiences and personal preferences. Empirical evidence from survey studies in Denmark suggests that bilateral trust between health professionals and individual patients is high (Enheden for brugerundersøgelser, 2009; Radiuskommunikation, 2016). This is also suggested indirectly by the continued high satisfaction rates among citizens who have received treatment in the health system (LUP, 2016).

Yet, at the same time, there are indications that trust may be reduced in regard to some aspects of system-level performance. A survey among 6,000 Danes in 2016 showed that trust was low in relation to the coordination of care. A majority of the respondents also lacked trust as regards expectations about receiving the right medicine and care. It is an important point that the respondents in this survey did not necessarily have personal experiences with the health system. In other words, the results reflect a more general perception within some parts of the population about the quality and service level of the health care system (Mandag Morgen and TrygFonden, 2016).

The reputational challenges of the public health care system are also a factor behind the growth in the number of citizens that hold private voluntary health insurance (Alexandersen et al, 2016). Although tax conditions and competition for skilled labour are part of the explanation, it seems clear that the reputation of public health organisations, particularly as regards waiting times and service quality, is another key factor. Summing up, it appears that patients continue to trust health professionals and that satisfaction is high among people who have actually used the public health system. Yet, at the same time, there seems to be an erosion of trust in the public health care system in general, and especially in its ability to cope with complex care issues.

Conclusion

This chapter has analysed developments in the regulation of health care and health professionals in Scandinavia. The importance of institutional features for regulation to promote the public interest has been highlighted. In particular, it has been argued that the high level of public involvement – with democratic management at state, region/ county and municipal levels – provides a structure in which to discuss different perceptions of the public interest. The regulation of health professionals has been analysed from a general system perspective and in regard to the role of patients in the regulatory process. We have observed that regulation is multidimensional but closely related to the highly public nature of Scandinavian health care systems. As such, we have seen that much regulation takes place in hierarchically connected accountability systems, and that employer-employee relations are at the core. However, this system for ongoing regulation is supplemented by external scrutiny by national authorities that have the power to issue and revoke licences and to intervene against individual health professionals.

Citizens/patients can influence health professionals in several ways. It is useful to distinguish between choice, voice and co-production mechanisms. A particularly important voice mechanism is the possibility of issuing formal complaints, which are then handled by regional and national-level authorities. Few cases are taken outside this system to be handled in the formal court system. All three of the Scandinavian countries examined in this chapter have extensive regulation of patients' rights – including access to information, informed consent and access to treatment. This legislation provides a basis for patient-professional interactions in the system. Patient/citizen voices are also heard through the governance of health care by democratic assemblies at several levels (local, regional and national).

Based on the analysis, we conclude that the formal conditions for pursuing the public interest are good, due to the democratic and public nature of the systems and the high level of transparency in decision making. This is also reflected in the high level of general trust in society. The level of trust between patients and professionals is also high. At the same time, there are some indications that the trust within the general population is lower than among citizens who have used the health system. Indications of reduced system-level trust can be seen in the growth in voluntary private health insurance (to bypass public providers), and in the relatively negative responses in national surveys about trust in the level of coordination within the system.

References

Alexandersen, N., Anell, A., Kaarboe, O., Lehto, J. S., Tynkkynen, L.-K. and Vrangbæk, K. (2016) 'The development of voluntary private health insurance in the Nordic countries', *Nordic Journal of Health Economics* 4(1): 68-83.

Bevan, G. and Hood, C. (2009) 'What's measured is what matters: targets and gaming in the English public health care system', *Public Administration* 84(3): 517-38.

Bovens, M. (2007) 'Analysing and assessing accountability: a conceptual framework', *European Law Journal* 13(4): 447-68.

Christiansen, T. and Vrangbæk, K. (2018, under review) 'Hospital centralization and performance in Denmark – ten years on', *Health Policy*.

Dent, M., Fallon, C., Wendt, C., Vuori, J., Puhor, M., de Pietro, C. and Silva, S. (2011) 'Medicine and user involvement within European healthcare: a typology for European comparative research', *International Journal of Clinical Practice* 65(12): 1218-20.

Dunston, R., Lee, A., Boud, D. and Chiarella, M. (2009) 'Co-production and health system reform – from re-imagining to re-making', *Australian Journal of Public Administration* 68(1): 39-58.

Enheden for brugerundersøgelser (2009) *Landsdækkende undersøgelse af kræftpatienters oplevelser*, København: Ministeriet for Sundhed og ForebyggelseHjelmar, U. and Hansen, S. W. (2013) *Lokalpolitik og borgere*, Copenhagen: KORA.

Jacobsen, C. B., Pedersen, V. H. and Albeck, K. (2008) 'Patientinddragelse mellem ideal og virkelighed – en empirisk undersøgelse af fælles beslutningstagning og dagligdagens møder mellem patient og behandler', in *Health Technology Assessment DSI Rapport*, Copenhagen: Sundhedsstyrelsen, Monitorering & Medicinsk Teknologivurdering og Dansk Sundhedsinstitut.

Klenk, T., Vrangbæk, K., Appleby, J. and Gregory, S. (2016) 'Accountability through performance management? Hospital performance management schemes in Denmark, Germany, and England', in Christensen, T. and Lægreid, P. (eds) *The Routledge Handbook of Accountability and Welfare State Reform in Europe*, London: Routledge.

LUP (2016) *Den Landsdækkende undersøgelse af patientoplevelser*, Frederiksberg, Denmark: Enhed for Evaluering og Brugerinddragelse, http://patientoplevelser.dk/files/dokumenter/filer/LUP/LUP2016/lup_2016_rapport.pdf

Magnussen, J., Vrangbæk, K., Saltman, R. B. (eds) (2009) *Nordic Health Care Systems: Recent Reforms and Current Policy Challenges*, Maidenhead: Open University Press.

Mandag Morgen and TrygFonden (2016) *Sundhedsvæsenet ifølge danskerne*, Copenhagen: Mandag Morgen and TrygFonden, Martin, H. M. (2010) *Er der styr på mig?*, Copenhagen: Dansk Sundhedsinstitut. www.kora.dk/media/1039630/er-der-styr-paa-mig.pdf

Obel, J. and Lintz, L. (2012) 'Kun en fjerdedel af lægernes tid bliver brugt med patienterne', *Politiken* 21 March, https://politiken.dk/debat/art5053079/Kun-en-fjerdedel-af-l%C3%A6gernes-tid-bliver-brugt-med-patienterne

Opedal, S., Rommetvedt, H. and Vrangbæk, K. (2012) 'Organized interests, authority structures and political influence: Danish and Norwegian patient groups compared', *Scandinavian Political Studies* 35(1): 1-21.

Øvretveit, J. (2003) 'Nordic privatization and private healthcare', *International Journal of Health Planning and Management* 18: 233-46.

Pedersen, L. and Kirk, K. (2014) 'Ny rolle – og magtfordeling mellem patienter og sundhedsprofessionelle – patient empowerment i teori og praksis', *Tidsskrift for Dansk Sundhedsvæsen* 90(2): 30-43.

Pestoff, V. (2012) 'Co-production and third sector social services in Europe: some crucial conceptual issues', in Pestoff, B., Brandsen, T. and Verschuere, B. (eds) *New Public Governance, the Third Sector and Co-production*, New York, NY: Routledge.

Radiuskommunikation (2016) 'Troværdighedsanalyse 2016: Mange faggrupper oplever stigende troværdighed', *Radius* 16 November, http://radiuskommunikation.dk/trovaerdighedsanalyse-2016-mange-faggrupper-oplever-stigende-trovaerdighed/

Rothstein, B. (2011) *The Quality of Government: Corruption, Social Trust, and Inequality in International Perspective*, Chicago, IL: University of Chicago Press.

Røvik, K. A. (1998) *Moderne organisasjoner: Trender i organisasjonstenkningen ved tusenårsskiftet*, Bergen: Fagbokforlaget.

Sahlin, K. and Wedlin, S. (2008) 'Circulating ideas: imitation, translation and editing', in Greenwood, R., Oliver, C., Suddaby, R. and Sahlin, K. (eds) *The SAGE Handbook of Organizational Institutionalism*, London: Sage.

Vrangbæk, K. (1999) *Markedsorientering i sygehussektoren*, Copenhagen: Institut for Statskundskab.

Vrangbæk, K. (2015) 'Patient involvement in Danish health care', *Journal of Health, Organization and Management* 29(5): 611-24.

Vrangbæk, K. (2017) 'Health systems of Scandinavia', in Cockerham, W. C. (ed) *International Encyclopedia of Public Health* (2nd edition), Oxford: Academic Press.

FIVE

Medical regulation for the public interest in the United Kingdom

William Roche

Introduction

The regulation of the medical profession encompasses three interrelated activities:

- the recognition of achievement of the required standard of education and training by potential doctors;
- the maintenance of a register of qualified doctors;
- the removal of doctors from such a register when issues of conduct or capability are found to be incompatible with continued registration.

While the public interest and the interests of the medical profession often coincide, such as in the case of the exclusion of unqualified persons from the register and the practice of medicine, there are times when the activity of regulation may be viewed as unduly lenient by the public or as too severe by the medical profession.

The current regulatory system in the United Kingdom (UK) has evolved over many years and its development has often been in response to crises in the confidence of either the public or elements of the medical profession. An understanding of the current system requires that its history is explored. It is evident that the General Medical Council (GMC), from its very beginnings, has attempted to achieve a balance in responding to concerns expressed by the public and those expressed by the profession. The relative sway of these sometime opposing forces has fluctuated with either being seen as the dominant influence at different times. For this reason, it is germane to consider a series of recent events and reports that have highlighted the expectations of the role of the GMC.

History

The ecclesiastical domination of many aspects of life in the Middle Ages that would be now regarded as secular extended to the recognition of physicians, the majority of whom were in holy orders. Ironically, the initial escape from religious control by the barber-surgeons can be traced to the 18th Canon of the Fourth Lateran Council in 1215, which banned clergy – including sub-deacons, deacons and priests – from being involved in the punitive shedding of blood and the practise of the art of surgery, which involves cauterising and making incisions (Fourth Lateran Council, 1215).

The surgeons proceeded to organise themselves through the guild system; the Barbers' Company was founded in 1308 and formally recognised in 1376 and the Fellowship of Surgeons was established in 1365 (Colson and Ralley, 2015). The Barbers' Company acquired royal patronage and received a Royal Charter in 1462. In 1540, King Henry VIII signed a charter incorporating barbers and surgeons by an Act of Parliament as the Guild of Barbers and Surgeons of London, which was the predecessor of the Royal College of Surgeons. A similar body was formed in Scotland in 1505 when the Barber Surgeons of Edinburgh was formally incorporated as a Craft Guild by the city authorities.

The physicians were also aware of the competition and perceived safety risks associated with unqualified practitioners. A small group of physicians led by Thomas Linacre petitioned King Henry VIII to establish a College of Physicians in 1518. This body evolved into the Royal College of Physicians of London during the 17th century, while in Edinburgh a Royal Charter was granted to the Royal College of Physicians in 1681. The London-based college required that fellows were graduates of Oxford or Cambridge, a duopoly that persisted until 1835, despite considerable unrest among its non-Oxbridge licentiates (Rivlin, 1997).

There was little evidence of the emergence of an all-encompassing medical profession, let alone one that was properly regulated. Interestingly, in 1423 there was an attempt to form an alliance between physicians and surgeons, the Conjoint College of Physicians and Surgeons, the chief architect of which was Gilbert Kymer, physician and vice-chancellor and later chancellor of Oxford University. The college was to regulate the apothecaries but they were not to be represented in its governance. The venture lasted a year and its one attempt to deal with alleged surgical malpractice foundered as a successful clinical outcome was regarded as unlikely due to malign astrological influences. There was a cross-professional initiative in Scotland in 1599, when

King James VI granted a Royal Charter to the Glasgow Faculty, which subsequently became the Royal College of Physicians and Surgeons of Glasgow, to control training and the professional activity of physicians, surgeons and dentists in the West of Scotland.

However, this system of regulation by the nascent Royal Colleges was of little relevance to the majority of the non-metropolitan population and to the less wealthy. For those who could afford any form of conventional medical treatment, the apothecary was the main source of assistance. Apothecaries were regarded as tradesmen and had been trained by apprenticeship rather than the classical Oxbridge education of the physicians. In addition to selling and dispensing medicine, they visited sick people at home and some apothecaries performed surgery. As access to the profession of apothecary was not limited to those who could afford a university education, they grew in number and were perceived as a threat, particularly by the physicians.

In the early 18th century, William Rose, a liveryman of the Society of Apothecaries, practising in the parish of St Martin-in-the-Fields, was prosecuted for practising medicine (Jones, 2006). The case was appealed to the House of Lords, where the arguments presented by the College of Physicians included the assertion that the practise of medicine by apothecaries would 'deprive the gentry of one of the professions by which their younger sons might honourably subsist and be a great detriment to the Universities' (Jones, 2006: 131). The Lords regarded the physicians' stance as being based on self-interest rather than the interest of patients and the public and allowed the appeal against the conviction of Rose in the case. In so doing, the Lords crystallised a criticism of the motivation of the medical profession in regulatory activity that is still heard three hundred years later. The finding also created, by precedent if not by legislation, legal recognition of the apothecary as a general medical practitioner. This development also had the unfortunate consequence of institutionalising the professional separation between the established bodies of physicians and surgeons and the general practitioners, a chasm that has continued to impact on the nature and provision of medical services in the UK.

While this feudal guild system benefited a medical and surgical elite, there is little evidence that it contributed to the wellbeing of the mass of the population. The regulation of the medical profession continued to be based on the descendants of the medieval colleges and guilds until 1815, when the professional divisions between the dispensing chemists and the apothecaries and concerns about the practise of medicine by the apprenticed-trained apothecaries culminated in the passage of an Act for Better Regulating the Practice of Apothecaries throughout

England and Wales 1815 (the Apothecaries Act) (Holloway, 1966). The Act introduced a compulsory apprenticeship, formal education and qualifications for apothecaries as well as legal duties related to dispensing. However, surgery was not part of the apothecaries' curriculum and many candidates also took the membership of the Royal College of Surgeons, to facilitate the full range of general practice.

The Apothecaries Act did not stop the clamour for reform of the regulation of the admission to the profession and of the practice of medicine in the UK (Holloway, 1966). Parliament continued to be petitioned for legislation with some 32 medical Bills being introduced prior to the passage of the Medical Act in 1858 (Roberts, 2009). The Medical Act 1858 established the General Council of Medical Education and Registration of the UK as a statutory body. The main provisions of the Act were to:

- set up the GMC and branch councils;
- establish a register, published annually;
- decide which qualifications were registrable;
- establish a disciplinary code;
- supervise examinations and be cognisant of courses of study;
- publish a pharmacopoeia;
- permit the recovery of fees;
- nominate offices and functions restricted to registered persons;
- abolish geographical restrictions on practice.

The proposed composition of the council represented a major shift from professional self-regulation to the recognition of a role for government and non-medical professionals in the governance of the medical profession. As initially proposed, the council was to be composed of 23 members: nine members nominated by the medical bodies, eight members nominated by universities with medical faculties and six members appointed nominally by the Queen, but on the advice of the government. These six appointed members were not to be college office-bearers and it was not mandatory for university appointees to be medically qualified. During its parliamentary progress, the Bill was amended so as to remove the restriction on the Crown appointment of college officers. Thus, it was theoretically possible for the majority membership of the council to be lay. However, the lobbying influence of the medical profession should never be underestimated. All the Crown appointments were medical men, including the president of the British Medical Association. The first meeting of the council appointed the president of the Royal College of Physicians of London, Sir Benjamin Brodie, as president of the council. Thus, the medical hegemony became institutionalised in the newly formed council.

The Medical Register was published in 1859 and this was an advance on the previous medical directories, which were based on self-reported medical qualifications. Now at least the literate public could assure themselves of the standing and qualifications of medical practitioners. A criticism of the Medical Act 1858 was the profusion of medical qualifications which it described, but did nothing to coordinate or simplify. For example, the qualifications of licentiates of the London Society of Apothecaries and the Apothecaries' Hall Dublin were included among the recognised qualifications to practise medicine in the UK. Although the apothecaries' bodies were examining and licensing bodies and not teaching organisations, their authority to grant recognised medical qualifications continued until the latter half of the 20th century, to the disquiet of some (Wakeford, 1987).

The next major legislative advance came with the Medical Act in 1950, which was based largely on recommendations of a committee chaired by the appositely named Sir William Goodenough (*British Medical Journal*, 1950). The 1950 Act renamed the General Council of Medical Education and Registration of the UK as the GMC. The Act provided for the establishment of a disciplinary committee with right of appeal to the judicial committee of the Privy Council either on points of law or on points of fact. The GMC was granted new powers to inspect the medical tuition afforded to students at medical schools, as hitherto the council only had powers to attend at examinations. A compulsory post-qualification training period was also introduced.

Key recent events and issues

The past three decades have been marked by a series of failings in the quality of health care on an organisational level, which have led to public and political questioning of the role and effectiveness of the GMC, as well as other regulatory bodies. At the same time, concerns have been expressed about the impact of regulatory processes on the wellbeing and survival of registrants under investigation. These parallel processes have been testing for the GMC, as they suggest underlying tendencies for leniency and for disproportionate severity in the discharge of its statutory duties.

Minority ethnic doctors and non-UK medical graduates

There have been persistent concerns that the GMC takes actions against a disproportionately high number of minority-ethnic doctors and non-UK medical graduates. The council considered reports from the Policy Studies Institute in 1996 and 2000 (Allen, 2000; Humphrey et al, 2009). The findings indicated that non-UK graduates were more likely to be referred to the GMC by complainants. The authors also reported inconsistency, poor recording and a lack of transparency of the GMC's processes in general. The GMC has continued to monitor these issues and to commission external reports. In 2014, there was no evidence of bias or discriminatory practices discovered and the investigators found decisions to be appropriate (de Bere et al, 2014). However, there was repetition of previous findings indicating a need for greater clarity and transparency in records of decision making. A related issue arose after a patient died following an accidental overdose of intravenous diamorphine that was administered by a locum out-of-hours general practitioner (GP) of German nationality who had previously failed a language assessment. The issue of competency in the English language has also been the subject of a recommendation in the report by Francis (2013) on the Mid Staffordshire NHS Foundation Trust. While the GMC required doctors from outside the European Union to undergo competence checks and English language tests, there was no such requirement for doctors from the European Economic Area. Following the outcry about this case, in 2014 the GMC gained powers to ensure that European doctors applying to work in the UK had recent evidence of their English language skills before being allowed a licence to practise.

The Bristol Royal Infirmary Inquiry

The Bristol Royal Infirmary Inquiry was set up in 1998 to investigate the deaths of 29 babies who underwent heart surgery at the hospital in the late 1980s and early 1990s (Kennedy, 2001). The GMC had held a long hearing into the conduct and performance of three doctors, the trust's chief executive, the medical director, the senior cardiac surgeon and another cardiac surgeon. All of the latter three were found guilty of serious professional misconduct for having continued to operate on children with unacceptably poor outcomes and for not intervening to stop the procedures. Two of the doctors were erased from the Medical Register and the third surgeon had conditions imposed on his registration, including a ban from operating on children for three years in the first instance. There were public protests at the decision not to erase the third surgeon and at the limited scope of the GMC's investigations. Criticism was voiced by the Secretary of State for Health, who ordered a public inquiry into cardiac surgery for children at the trust. The public confidence in the GMC and the concept of professional self-regulation was severely damaged. Among its many recommendations, the Kennedy report into the scandal at the hospital urged the requirement for regular appraisal, the revalidation of medical practitioners and better local investigation and management of issues related to registered health care professionals.

The Shipman Inquiry

Dr Harold Shipman, the UK's worst serial killer, was jailed in January 2000 for killing 15 of his patients, but it is thought that he murdered some 250 in total. He had already been subject to the attention of the GMC because of concerns about his abuse of opiates, although there were more pertinent procedural failings that prevented the earlier detection of his crimes. The GP was given 15 life sentences for the murders, committed by administering fatal doses of diamorphine. The Shipman Inquiry, led by Dame Janet Smith, produced six reports on the doctor's crimes, the fifth of which dealt with regulatory and disciplinary procedures (Smith, 2004). Dame Janet was critical of the GMC as being overprotective of doctors and the chief medical officer, Sir Liam Donaldson, was even more forthright (DH, 2006). Donaldson echoed concerns about the GMC's fitness to practise (FtP) procedures and other functions of the council. In his view, complaints were dealt with in a haphazard manner, and the GMC caused distress to doctors over trivial complaints while tolerating poor practice in other cases. He echoed the view that 'for members of the public or those taking a public interest perspective, the concern has been that medical regulatory processes have been too secretive, too tolerant of sub-standard practice and too dominated by the professional interest, rather than that of the patient' (Smith, 2004: 11). Dame Janet had criticisms and recommendations about practically every aspect of the GMC's FtP procedures, the most salient of which was the recommendation to separate the adjudication stage of these procedures and have the functions performed by a body independent of the GMC.

The Mid Staffordshire Hospital

There was a public outcry at the poor care and excessive mortality between 2005 and 2009 at the Mid Staffordshire Hospital, a small district general hospital in the Midlands in England. A report was published of the public inquiry, chaired by Robert Francis QC, into the regulatory and other failings that allowed the persistent poor care at the Mid Staffordshire NHS Foundation Trust (Francis, 2013). Among the 290 recommendations, Francis urged:

- openness, transparency and candour throughout the health care system (including a statutory duty of candour);
- fundamental standards for health care providers better cooperation between regulators of professional standards and regulators of health care provision.

Again, there was public discontent at the decision of the GMC not to proceed against the medical managers of the trust, despite the finding that there had been a failure of senior leadership.

Deaths of doctors under investigation

It is generally recognised that medical professionals have a higher risk of completed suicide than the general population. Although some individual incidents of suicide of doctors while under investigation by the GMC had attracted attention, an internal report commissioned by the GMC found that 28 doctors who were subject to GMC processes had died as a result of suicide or suspected suicide between 2005 and 2013 (Horsfall, 2014). Of these 28 doctors, 20 had health concerns but only in six (30%) of the 20 health concern cases was a specific risk of suicide known to the GMC. This high mortality rate led the GMC to commission a support service from the British Medical Association for doctors with whom there was FtP involvement.

Postgraduate medical education

Prior to 2010, postgraduate medical education was governed by a quasi-independent public body, the Postgraduate Medical Education and Training Board. There was a view in the profession that this board was neither effective nor cooperative with the medical Royal Colleges. Professor Sir John Tooke led an independent inquiry into the structure and delivery of postgraduate medical education and recommended that the GMC absorb the regulatory function related to the completion of postgraduate training (Tooke, 2008). This occurred in April 2010 and led to the GMC overseeing the continuum of undergraduate and postgraduate medical education and training. It is interesting to reflect that this outcome was recommended as early as 1975 in the Merrison report (Douglas, 1975).

Current legislation and regulatory functions

The current legislative basis for the GMC is the Medical Act of 1983 and its subsequent amendments and Statutory Orders of the Privy Council, which include the approval of changes made in the regulations by the GMC. The 1983 Act defines the purpose of the council, its governance structure and its statutory purpose of the regulation of medical education, and admission to and removal from the professional register, and the provision of guidance on professional performance, conduct and ethics. An important additional role was enshrined in the Medical (Professional Performance) Act 1995, which empowers the GMC to deal with underperforming doctors in addition to doctors accused of misconduct. Of particular note is section 60 of the Health Act 1999. This allows the Department of Health to introduce changes to primary legislation related to professional regulation by means of an Order through the Privy Council, although there is a requirement for consultation and Parliament may review the responses to any such consultation. This facility has been used to reform the processes of tribunal hearings into allegations against doctors.

Representation on the General Medical Council

The structure of the GMC as initially constituted under the 1983 Act reflected some of the concerns about public accountability that initially influenced the structure of the council, which was proposed in the Medical Act 1858. A council of 104 members included three categories of council members, defined as 54 elected members, 25 appointed members and 25 nominated members. The elected members were registered doctors elected by their fellow doctors on the register every five years from four constituencies: England, the Channel Islands and the Isle of Man, Northern Ireland, Scotland and Wales. Appointed members were registered doctors appointed by universities with medical schools and by the Royal Colleges and their faculties. Nominated members were Crown appointments on the advice of the Privy Council. These were the lay members, selected from the establishment and confined to a small minority of the 104 members.

This GMC structure was subject to a number of criticisms, including the bloated number of its members and its consequential unwieldy processes and the overwhelming medical majority. In 2003, the membership of the council was reduced from 104 members to 35 and the proportion of lay members was increased from 24% to 40%. It was not until 2012 that the Department of Health recommended that the council was reduced to 12 members with 50% lay members. Appointment to membership of the council became a selection procedure with assessment against a competency framework, with the chair also being selected through a similar process rather than being elected. Although members of the council are strictly not representatives, at least one member must live or work wholly or mainly in each of England, Wales, Northern Ireland and Scotland.

The function of the council is to act in a manner analogous to the board of a company. It is required to ensure that the GMC is properly managed by the chief executive, whom it holds to account for the performance of the council against its statutory and charitable purposes to protect, promote and maintain the health and safety of the public by ensuring proper standards in the practice of medicine. The GMC also has charitable status and council members act as the trustees of the registered charity.

Accountability

The GMC has to negotiate a complex series of relationships with the public, the medical profession, government and Parliament. The drafting of legislation that gives the GMC its authority and defines its functions is the duty of the English Department of Health. However, the GMC is not accountable to the Department of Health nor to the UK government. Instead, it reports to Parliament, via the Health Committee. Unusually for an organisation with such accountability, the activities of the GMC are funded from the fees that it raises from registered doctors and which it levies for examinations and assessments. While there is no statutory accountability to the profession, the GMC can only function as an effective regulator if it maintains the confidence of the medical profession. As the GMC has increasingly recognised its public duties, this has caused some doctors to express disquiet at the situation whereby they fund an organisation the primary duty of which is to act for the public benefit and on which they have no elected representation.

In contrast, a series high-profile failings in health care provider organisations and in the practice of individual doctors, as noted earlier, has led to an increasing clamour in the media for reform of the GMC. The views expressed include the contention that the GMC protects doctors rather than the public, which is directly contrary to the concerns expressed by some doctors. This highlights the conflicting expectations of its various stakeholders, which can change abruptly when an individual becomes the victim of perceived malpractice or comes under regulatory scrutiny.

Revalidation

Prior to 2012, the majority of doctors had no contact with the GMC apart from their initial registration and notice of their annual subscription. This often continued until their demise as many doctors, for reasons of emotional attachment or for the sake of convenience, maintained their registration beyond their retirement. This relationship changed fundamentally when, in response to the public and political pressure arising from the scandalous failings in the 1990s and 2000s, revalidation was introduced in December 2012. The concept of regular review of a doctor's freedom to practise medicine had been mooted since the 1970s, but adverse criticism of the GMC as a regulator in public reports finally spurred the GMC into action (Chamberlain, 2015).

Although the regular re-examination of a doctor's competencies, as recommended in the Shipman Inquiry, was rejected, doctors who wish to maintain their licence to practise medicine in the UK must now demonstrate that they are up to date and fit to practise. In this regard, revalidation is a step change in medical regulation as it aims to give positive assurance that doctors are safe to practise, rather than just ratifying the historical record of their qualification. Doctors are required to engage in regular appraisals and to produce evidence of participation, activity and reflection in four domains that have been distilled from the GMC's Good Medical Practice standards:

- knowledge, skills and performance;
- safety and quality;
- communication, partnership and teamwork;
- maintaining trust.

The revalidation structure is hierarchical, with practically every licenced doctor connected to a designated body that has a medical responsible officer, who is usually the medical director of that organisation. These responsible officers are themselves connected to a level two responsible officer within the NHS hierarchy, even if they are not performers of NHS work. There are other ways of connecting for doctors who do not hold clinical contracts or who do not fit into the hierarchy described. Thus, all licenced doctors should have a relationship with a senior doctor who can monitor their ongoing FtP. This practice includes all aspects of the doctor's regulated activity, not just that which is performed on behalf of their main employer. Every five years, the responsible officer makes a recommendation to the GMC about the revalidation of the licences of the doctors with whom they are connected. Each responsible officer has the ability to discuss matters with a regional GMC employer liaison adviser. This is a significant change from the situation whereby the only contact with the GMC was as a referral of concerns about a doctor. The role of the employer liaison adviser allows for the exchange of information about performing doctors and advice on threshold and mechanisms for dealing with concerns.

In 2017, Sir Keith Pearson reported on the first four years of revalidation (Pearson, 2017). He found that the process had been met with general acceptance by the profession, had increased compliance with appraisals, albeit more in terms of frequency than content, and had strengthened governance in organisations. However, there was a lack of public understanding of the process and how the public and patients might engage in feedback on a doctor's performance. Health care provider organisations also needed to develop ways in which to provide more timely information to doctors on their performance. Although the system had improved the appraisal of locum doctors, there was more to be done to improve their appraisals and assessment. Perhaps because the events that precipitated the introduction of revalidation led to a focus on poor performance and behaviours, the senior medical leadership has yet to voice enthusiasm for the potential role of this process as a key tool to deliver improvements in patients' experience of care and in the quality of clinical outcomes for all doctors.

Fitness to practise procedures

The investigation and adjudication of complaints and concerns about doctors is an essential corollary of the maintenance of a register of doctors who are fit to practise medicine. However, there has been repeated criticism of the GMC for combining the roles of investigation, prosecution and adjudication. Following Dame Janet Smith's criticisms in the Shipman report (2004), the Medical Practitioners Tribunal Service (MPTS) was established in June 2012, with the aim of providing a clear separation between the GMC's investigation function and the adjudication of hearings (Chamberlain, 2015). In March 2015, the Privy Council approved a section 60 Order amending the Medical Act 1983. This further separated the MPTS from the GMC by placing it on a statutory footing rather than solely as a committee of the GMC. FtP panels and interim orders panels thereafter became known as medical practitioners tribunals and interim orders tribunals.

Complaints and concerns are reviewed by the GMC, at which stage it may dismiss the complaint or make preliminary inquiries with the doctor's employer or responsible officer. If an investigation appears to be warranted, this may include the gathering of evidence, witness statements and expert reports on clinical matters. The GMC may also order assessments of the doctor's performance, their health or their knowledge of the English language. At the end of the investigation, two case examiners (one medical and one non-medical) may decide to dismiss the case, issue a warning, agree undertakings on health and performance issues following a health or performance assessment or refer the case to the MPTS for a tribunal hearing. If the case examiners cannot reach a consensus, the case is referred to the Investigation Committee, a statutory committee of the GMC that determines the next step. The Investigation Committee also reviews cases where the doctor does not accept the findings and decision of the case examiners to issue a warning. In such cases, the Investigation Committee sits in public.

The case examiners of the Investigation Committee are required to apply a 'realistic prospect' test to the alleged facts to determine whether they are likely to be found proven and, if so established, whether the facts would be sufficiently grave to demonstrate that the practitioner's FtP is impaired to a degree justifying action on their registration. While the case examiners are required to assess the weight of the evidence, they should not attempt to address substantial conflicts of evidence. In addition, they are supposed to take cognisance of any prior decision made by another public body with medical input into the matter. At any stage in the proceedings, the GMC may refer the doctor to the MPTS for an interim orders tribunal hearing if it appears that it may be necessary for the protection of members of the public, in the public interest or in the interests of the doctor, to act immediately on their registration. As well as the protection of the public, the public interest includes preserving public trust in the profession and maintaining good standards of conduct and performance. An interim orders tribunal can suspend or restrict a doctor from practising while the investigation continues. However, such actions are not intended to influence the outcome of any subsequent tribunal hearing.

An MPTS tribunal consists of three tribunalists drawn from specially trained doctors and members of the public, who hear the evidence and find on facts based on the 'civil standard of proof' – that is, whether the facts were more likely to have occurred than not. Prior to adopting the civil standard of proof in 2008, the GMC required the 'criminal standard of proof' – that is, whether the facts occurred 'beyond reasonable doubt'. The tribunal then determines whether the facts mean that the doctor's FtP is impaired and, if so, what sanction, if any, should be applied. Hearings are held in public, unless the tribunal is hearing confidential evidence about a doctor's health. The determinations, including the reasons for the findings and the actions taken, are published on the MPTS website. The sanctions available to a tribunal that finds a doctor's FtP to be impaired include:

- placing restrictive conditions on the doctor's registration;
- suspension from the Medical Register, so that the doctor cannot practise during the period of suspension;
- erasure of the doctor from the Medical Register.

There is a public perception that erasure from the register is final and irrevocable. However, a doctor can apply for restoration to the register five years or more after the date of erasure. A restoration application is heard by an MPTS tribunal that requires evidence that the doctor has achieved insight into the issues that led to erasure and has remedied these. In addition, the doctor must demonstrate that their medical knowledge and skills are up to date and that it is safe for them to resume practice.

Appeals against tribunal decisions

There are rights of appeal to the High Court against a final decision made by an MPTS tribunal the GMC or the Professional Standards Authority for Health and Social Care. The Professional Standards Authority reviews the decisions of the FtP tribunals or panels of nine health care regulators in the UK and has the right under section 29 of the NHS Reform and Health Care Professions Act 2002 to refer a medical practitioner tribunal decision to the relevant court if it believes that it is not sufficient for the protection of the public. In 2015, the GMC also acquired the power to refer MPTS decisions for review where it regards the sanction imposed as inadequate for public protection. On appeal, a judge can allow or dismiss the appeal, or substitute for the sanction or order appealed against with any other variation that could have been given by the panel, or pass the case to the registrar of the GMC to refer it to a medical practitioner tribunal to deal with it in accordance with the directions of the court.

However, there is no mechanism of appeal against a decision of the GMC not to proceed to investigate a case or to refer it to the MPTS for adjudication. This is an area of ongoing contention, as reflected in the responses to the Mid Staffordshire and Bristol scandals. The requirement that the case examiners or Investigation Committee should state the reasons for any decision that may be perceived to be inconsistent with a decision made by an NHS trust, coroner or ombudsman seems to be neither well recognised nor met comprehensively in practice. While it must be acknowledged that there are restrictions due to the peril of being found to have defamed a registrant where the facts have not been found by the GMC, better communication of the reasons for not acting would serve to enhance the public perception of the accountability of the GMC, particularly in cases with a high profile in the media.

Conclusion

As this chapter has demonstrated, the regulation of the medical profession in the UK has a long and complex history. Reform has often been driven by public outcry, frequently directed against the perceived hegemony of the profession. It is almost certain that the twin forces of professional and public opinion will continue to drive the evolution of medical regulation in the UK. There is a gradual movement to ensure the greater involvement of the public at all levels of regulatory activity. The challenge for the GMC is to bring the medical profession with it in this journey to achieve greater openness and accountability.

References

Allen, I. (2000) *The Handling of Complaints by the GMC: A Study of Decision-Making and Outcomes*, London: Policy Studies Institute.

British Medical Journal (1950) 'The Medical Act, 1950', *British Medical Journal* 2(4674): 337–8.

Chamberlain, J. M. (2015) *Medical Regulation, Fitness to Practise and Revalidation*, Bristol: Policy Press.

Colson, J. and Ralley, R. (2015) 'Medical practice, urban politics and patronage: the London "commonalty" of physicians and surgeons of the 1420s', *English Historical Review* 130(546): 1102–31.

de Bere, S. R., Bryce, M., Archer, J., Nunn S., Lynn N. and Roberts, M. (2014) *Review of Decision-Making in the General Medical Council's Fitness to Practise Procedures*, Plymouth: University of Plymouth.

DH (Department of Health) (2006) *Good Doctors, Safer Patients: Proposals to Strengthen the System to Assure and Improve the Performance of Doctors and to Protect the Safety of Patients*, report by the chief medical officer, London: DH.

Douglas, C. P. (1975) 'Report of the Merrison Committee', *Proceedings of the Royal Society of Medicine* 68(11): 763.

Fourth Lateran Council (1215) *Fourth Lateran Council: 1215*, www.papalencyclicals.net/Councils/ecum12-2.htm

Francis, R. (2013) *Report of the Mid Staffordshire NHS Foundation Trust Public Inquiry*, London: The Stationery Office.

Holloway, S. W. F. (1966) 'The Apothecaries Act, 1815: a reinterpretation', *Medical History* 10(2): 107-29.

Horsfall, S. (2014) *Doctors who Commit Suicide while under GMC Fitness to Practise Investigation*, London: General Medical Council.

Humphrey, C. et al (2009) *Clarifying the Factors Associated with Progression of Cases in the GMC's Fitness to Practise Procedures: Full Research Report*, Swindon: Economic and Social Research Council.

Jones, R. (2006) 'Apothecaries, physicians and surgeons', *British Journal of General Practice* 56(524): 232-3.

Kennedy, I. (2001) *The Report of the Public Inquiry into Children's Heart Surgery at the Bristol Royal Infirmary 1984-1995: Learning from Bristol*, Cm5207, London: The Stationery Office.

Pearson, K. (2017) *Taking Revalidation Forward: Improving the Process of Relicensing for Doctors*, London: General Medical Council.

Rivlin, J. J. (1997) 'Getting a medical qualification in England in the nineteenth century', *Medical Historian* 9: 56-63.

Roberts, M. J. D. (2009) 'The politics of professionalization: MPs, medical men, and the 1858 Medical Act', *Medical History* 53(1): 37-56.

Smith, J. (2004) *The Shipman Inquiry: Fifth Report: Safeguarding Patients: Lessons from the Past – Proposals for the Future*, Cm 6394, London: The Stationery Office.

Tooke, J. (2008) *Aspiring to Excellence: Final Report of the Independent Inquiry into Modernising Medical Careers*, London: MMC Inquiry

Wakeford, R. (1987) 'LMSSA: a back door entry into medicine?', *British Medical Journal* 294(6575): 890-1.

SIX

Regulating the regulators: the rise of the United Kingdom Professional Standards Authority

Judith Allsop and Kathryn Jones

Introduction

For the past two decades, the way in which health professionals are regulated has undergone major evolutionary change. There have been inquiries, reports, new legislation, changes in practice and new institutions. The traditional form of self-regulation has given way to appointed professional councils that regulate professionals across nine professions, which since 2002 have been overseen by a meta-regulator. The Professional Standards Authority for Healthcare and Social Care (PSA), previously named the Council for Health Regulatory Excellence (CHRE), regulates the regulators in the United Kingdom (UK). Since 2012, their remit has extended to social work, as well as the health care professions. The PSA is an 'arm's-length' agency of the Department of Health, England. A recent report from the Law Commission (2014) proposes further change. From the onset of the reforms, the aim has been to protect people who use professional services by ensuring safe practice although regulation also has an impact on the professionals who provide these services.

In this chapter we aim to describe and analyse the reform process. We look at the special case of regulating professional work, the underlying changes that created a case for reform, and the events that led to government action. We then clarify our understanding of 'regulation', and give an account of the reforms beginning in 2002 with the establishment of the meta-regulator. We go on to describe the changes in the structure of the professional councils following from the Health and Social Care Act 2008, which introduced a corporate form of governance, and an expansion of activity. Finally, we assess the outcome of reforms and the case for further change.

In order to assess the outcome of the reforms, we draw on data collected in 2004, when we were commissioned by the CHRE to undertake a scoping study of the nine regulatory councils (Allsop et al, 2004). Data were collected using a template pro-forma, which was completed by council officers. This covered their founding legislation, the structure of governance and selected indicators on resources and activity. In addition, we documented their role in:

- keeping a register of professionals;
- setting standards for education and practice;
- responding to complaints from the public through investigation to establish whether a professional's practice was impaired;
- adjudication by a panel to determine what action to take.

The process is referred to as fitness to practise (FtP). For this chapter, we collected comparative data for 2014/15 on the meta-regulator and the councils, from websites, reports and other documentary sources, to show the changes in activity and costs as well as developments in regulatory practice. This allows us to assess outcomes.

Why regulatory reform?

In most countries, the practice of health professionals is regulated. Their expertise is highly valued and sought after by the public and patients who want good-quality care. The model for professional regulation, in English-speaking countries in particular, has been state-licenced, self-regulation. With the Medical Act 1858, a regulatory bargain was struck between the state and the medical profession. Medical practitioners were registered as qualified by the General Medical Council (GMC). When the GMC was established, it was an organisation of its time. It was composed of elected members and allowed medical men to draw a boundary around their practice and exclude the unqualified. Doctors could display their registration status by title, and the public could identify them by this means. The GMC had disciplinary powers to exclude those 'who brought the profession into disrepute' and the state could keep a distance. This model was later extended to other health professions.

Although the language has changed, and the scope of functions expanded, professional councils now carry out similar core functions:

- they set standards for competence, behaviour and education;
- they maintain a register of those deemed fit to practise;
- they deal with the concerns raised by patients, the public and others where there is a fear that standards have not been met due ill-health, misconduct or poor performance – the FtP process.

What have been reformed are the role of state institutions and the governance structure of the professions.

Pressures for change have been due to multiple factors. Rapid advances in expert knowledge and techniques now require that professionals keep up to date with periodic reassessment. It is known that health care interventions carry a risk of avoidable adverse events and there are unacceptable variations in quality (Donaldson, 2000), as a senior doctor commented: 'Medicine used to be simple, ineffective and relatively safe. Now it is complex, effective and potentially dangerous' (GMC, 2000: 8). Patient safety and the prevention of harm have become a priority in many areas of public policy, especially in the health and social care sector. At the same time, demands on health care have increased and so has the propensity of the public to 'name' and 'claim' through making a complaint (Felstiner et al, 1981). The rise can be attributed to various interrelated factors such as:

- higher public expectations;
- better-educated consumers;
- consumer group activity;
- media coverage;
- an ageing population with complex needs
  (de Bere et al, 2014; GDC, 2014).

Over the past 20 years, well-publicised cases of serial poor performance, and inappropriate and sometimes criminal behaviour by health professionals, led to a number of inquiries. Extensive media coverage fuelled criticisms that were longstanding. Professional regulation was portrayed as self-serving and as failing to protect the public from harm. Inquiries opened up the opaque internal processes of professional councils to public scrutiny (for a forensic analysis, see Smith, 2004). They revealed a lack of due process for handling complaints and a lack of coordination between regulatory agencies to deal with poor practice. The details of these inquiries and the case for regulatory change are summarised in a report by the Department of Health (DH, 2007a). Within the medical profession, internal reforms were attempted but failed. This was initially due to disunity within the profession on the need for reform (Irvine, 2003) and, later, to a lack of consensus on proposals for the periodic revalidation of doctors' competence (Salter, 2007; Fenton and Salter, 2009).

The most compelling factor in triggering regulatory reform was that the existing system was seen as not fit for purpose by government and a number of other influential constituencies. Pressure for reform had come from patients and consumer bodies, from academia, from the elite lawyers who led the public inquiries, as well as from within the medical profession. While the underlying causes were social and technological, the final factor that enabled reform was a shift in the politics of professional regulation. Concerns about poor practice in nursing and midwifery that were later to conclude with the reports by Francis (2013) and Kirkup (2015) were beginning to surface and underlined the necessity for change.

It was also becoming apparent to the Department of Health that a number of occupational groups in health care were emerging who provided treatment, care and support in public and domestic settings. Some groups sought the status and identity afforded by statutory regulation; for others there was a concern about the lack of oversight (Saks and Allsop, 2007). The process of the professionalisation of occupational groups within the health and social care sector had expanded the workforce. By 2016, there were 1.44 million health and social care professionals regulated by one of the nine professional councils (PSA, 2016a).

What is regulation and how has it changed?

Drawing on Black (2002), we define regulation as a set of rules made by a superior authority to oversee another agency. The rules made are a focused and sustained attempt to alter the behaviour of others according to defined standards or purposes. Regulation is not an end in itself but aims to ensure that the agencies act in the public interest for the good of the community in a cost–effective way. Setting standards and ensuring compliance are part of the task.

Regulations are initiated by the government and neoliberal ideas about New Public Management (NPM) have led to the devolution of regulatory tasks to arm's-length agencies or external regulators (Flynn, 2012). Central governments 'steer' rather than 'row' (Day and Klein, 1997). In UK health care there are multiple agencies that have a role in setting the professional standards to determine and support good practice. The regulatory environment is complex, with separate and sometimes overlapping responsibilities between agencies. Professional councils only set the framework for practice and, in the case of the larger councils, have oversight over many thousands of registrants. The task becomes possible only if regulation is seen as a matrix of formal and informal controls. These range from the professional regulatory body to other regulators, professional associations, employers, specialist support bodies (such as the National Clinical Assessment Service) and quality and standards agencies (such as the Care Quality Commission). Professional regulation is about overseeing the relationship between the professional and the patient to ensure that professional norms and values continue to be internalised and are reinforced through colleague networks. The guidelines for practice issued by the professional body help professionals to negotiate difficult ethical and legal problems.

These developments have led Black (2002) to suggest that regulation has become 'decentred' from the state. Lower-level bodies are expected to identify problems and seek solutions. Effective regulation is a product of their interaction. Yet agencies are likely to have different powers, priorities and sources of information. Information sharing has proved to be difficult to achieve. For example, the report by Francis (2013) on the Inquiry into the longstanding abuse of patients at Mid Staffordshire NHS Foundation Trust noted that even within the same organisation, information that could have prevented the abuse was not shared.

Government committees have advised on the principles of regulation. For instance, the Better Regulation Task Force (2003) recommended transparency, accountability, consistency, proportionality and targeting. Identifying and targeting risks in order to increase safety has become popular, with comparisons made between health care and the aircraft industry. Although this appears a rational approach, some are sceptical. Hutter (2005) points out that there is no consistent definition of techniques for managing risk. Hood and colleagues (2001) have argued that there are difficulties in identifying risk in a situation where qualitative judgements are made, such as in the context of a professional–client relationship. These reservations are borne out by the analysis by Lloyd-Bostock and Hutter (2008) of the GMC's database on complaints and whether it could be used to assess risk factors. They concluded that it was inadequate for anticipating and prioritising risk factors. The data had been collected for a different purpose, associations between variables did not establish causality, and if used to take action could undermine relations between doctors and patients.

Reforming professional regulation: an evolutionary process

In the event, the reform of professional regulation has proceeded in a piecemeal fashion. For clarity, we divide it chronologically into three phases using particular Acts of Parliament as markers. The first phase can be taken from the NHS Reform and Health Professions Act 2002; the second from the Health and Social Care Act 2008; and the third from the Health and Social Care Act 2012. The Law Commission (2014) has proposed further changes to be incorporated in the Regulation of Health and Social Care Professions Etc. Bill (House of Lords, 2016). This heavy reliance on legislation to achieve reform illustrates the barriers to realising a shift in organisational cultures that are deeply embedded.

The introduction of a meta-regulator

The NHS Reform and Health Professions Act 2002 set up the CHRE and announced the intention to reform regulation for all the health professions. The CHRE was an arm's-length agency of the Department of Health, with a remit to work in the public interest and promote best practice. It was to act as a meta-regulator of the nine separate statutory health professional councils:

- General Chiropractic Council (GCC);
- General Dental Council (GDC);
- General Medical Council (GMC);
- General Optical Council (GOC);
- General Osteopathic Council (GOsC);
- Health Professions Council (HPC; after 2012 the Health and Care Professions Council [HCPC]);
- Nursing and Midwifery Council (NMC);
- Pharmaceutical Society of Northern Ireland (PSNI);
- Royal Pharmaceutical Society of Great Britain (RPS; after 2010 the General Pharmaceutical Council [GPhC]).

It also aimed to promote public understanding of regulation by consulting with patients, the public and other key stakeholders (CHRE, 2004).

The CHRE had a large board made up of 19 appointed members, of whom nine were the presidents of the aforementioned councils. The councils were to be reviewed annually for an assessment of how they carried out their functions. The aim was to encourage consistency in process and best regulatory practice through cooperation between the councils. The CHRE also had a specific power to scrutinise the outcome of decisions of individual councils in their FtP cases and, if they considered a sanction to be too lenient, under section 29 of the NHS Reform and Health Professions Act 2002 could refer a case to the High Court for further consideration. There was a perception at the time that some councils imposed harsher sanctions than others and that a further appeal stage was required to ensure that panel findings and outcomes were in the public interest.

For the first time, professional councils had a forum to discuss shared problems. An early decision was to undertake a scoping study of roles and functions, as little was known about the internal processes of each council (Allsop et al, 2004). Workshops run by the Department of Health used mixed breakout groups to discuss regulatory issues. From participant observation at the time, the authors' view is that some council leaders welcomed the opportunity to share common problems, while others did not.

Over the next few years, three reports indicated the determination of the government to proceed with reform:

- *Good Doctors, Safer Patients* (DH, 2006a);
- *The Regulation of Non-Medical Healthcare Professions* (DH, 2006b);
- *Safeguarding Patients: The Government's Response to the Recommendations of the Shipman Inquiry's Fifth Report* (DH, 2007a).

The subsequent White Paper (DH, 2007b) set the policy direction with the Health and Social Care Act 2008. The Inquiry by Francis (2013) into the abuse of patients in the Mid Staffordshire NHS Foundation Trust, and the report by Kirkup (2015) into failings in maternity services in Morecambe Bay, demonstrated systemic weaknesses. The latter report ended locally based arrangements for the regulation of midwives, bringing them fully under the regulatory umbrella of the Nursing and Midwifery Council (NMC). Both reports emphasised the importance of using information to identify, analyse and act on risk and urged regulators to cooperate with each other more closely to avoid harm to patients.

The Health and Social Care Act 2008 and its consequences

Following the Health and Social Care Act 2008, the CHRE was given a stronger strategic role in regulating professional councils with a pared-down corporate governance structure. The board consisted of seven publicly appointed members, four of whom had experience of the countries within the UK, and the chief executive. Professional councils were not represented. Its purpose was restated: its role was to promote the health, safety and wellbeing of patients and other members of the public and to be a strong, independent voice for patients throughout the UK, as well as a centre of regulatory expertise internationally. The powers of the CHRE were extended to include an overview of all stages of the investigation process as well as decisions made about ill-health or discipline. Harry Cayton, who had experience both in the health voluntary sector and as a watchdog for patients in government, was appointed as chief executive. In 2012, when the CHRE was renamed the Professional Standards Authority (PSA), he retained the post.

The regulatory role of professional councils was restated under the 2008 Act. This was to ensure the competence and skills of their registrants in order to protect the public. Councils became smaller with a board of 12 and 14 members appointed by government and with least parity between the lay and professional members. The board's role was to determine strategy. Accountability upwards was increased as councils were not only reviewed by the CHRE, but also accountable to Parliament through an annual hearing before the Health Select Committee. In practice, accountability hearings to date have only been held regularly with the GMC, the General Dental Council (GDC) and the NMC. Transcripts from these meetings are made available by the Health Select Committee on their website. This increases transparency.

The Act also established the Office of the Health Professions Adjudicator (OHPA). This followed the legal principle that there should be a separation between the body that investigates a case and the panel adjudicates. The OHPA was to take over the final stage of the FtP panel, initially for GMC and General Optical Council (GOC) cases. However, the OHPA was short-lived. In 2012, following a change in government, it was abolished. Instead, the government's preferred option was to 'enhance the independence of adjudication and modernise processes' (*Pharmaceutical Journal*, 2010). In the same year, the GMC established the Medical Practitioners Tribunal Service (MPTS). The tribunal is located in Manchester and the chair is a legally qualified judge.

Within the CHRE/PSA, regulatory processes follow principles of the Better Regulation Task Force with the addition of 'agility': anticipating change rather than responding to the last crisis (PSA, 2015a). Standards have sharpened and the agency has a higher public profile. The meta-regulator invites feedback from consumer organisations. Cayton now sees its role as not so much a regulator as 'an oversight and audit body'. It does not manage regulators or apply sanctions, but rather 'reviews and comments on what they are doing in order to raise standards' (comments to the Law Commission, 2014: 202). The concept of 'right-touch' regulation has been promoted (PSA, 2015b). This is seen as the minimum regulatory force necessary to achieve a result, taking risk into account. Risk may relate to the inherent dangers of an intervention, the context it takes place in, and the vulnerability or autonomy of the user.

Since 2010, the CHRE and then the PSA have published a comprehensive and specific set of standards, 24 in all, under the headings of their main functions. Each regulator is interrogated on how they meet these, backed up by evidence. Regulators submit evidence on the impact of their work in maintaining public confidence in the profession and are given examples as guidance. The meta-regulator then makes a collective judgement on the strengths and weaknesses in processes, and states what constitutes best practice. The methodology ensures that the standard is a moving one and weaknesses are identified and become part of the following year's review. There are also checks on a council's claims. For example, spot-checks can be made of the registers and onsite audits undertaken. In 2011, CHRE audits of the register of the NMC and of the FtP processes of both the NMC and GOC led to a detailed report in which both were criticised for being well below the standard required (CHRE, 2012).

The CHRE/PSA's annual report is publicly available and states whether each council has met, or failed to meet, a particular standard. The 2014/15 report says that only the HCPC, the GMC and the GOsC met all the standards while six of the nine regulators either did not meet, or were inconsistent on, one or more (PSA, 2015a). A detailed report for each council is specific about weaknesses so there is an element of 'naming' and 'shaming'. Kagan (1989: 92) identifies a range of options for regulators, on a spectrum from coercion and conciliation to cooperation. The style of the CHRE/PSA could be said to be focused and supportive. Councils are encouraged to innovate providing this protects patient safety but they are process focused and have no powers of enforcement or resources to solve problems. We do not know what councils themselves think about the regulatory style. The meta-regulator itself admits that it has few sanctions.

The PSA expands its role

By 2011 it had become clear that the regulatory reform was far from complete. The Department of Health published its strategy for regulating health professionals and asked the Law Commission to make proposals for further reform (DH, 2011). The Health and Social Care Act 2012 had renamed the meta-regulator as the PSA. This brought an expansion in jurisdiction. The PSA took over powers from the Privy Council to oversee appointments of the chair and the members of professional councils. It also began to regulate social workers in England and now accredits the voluntary registers of other groups of health care workers. By 2015, the PSA oversaw 18 voluntary registers and covered 32 professions (PSA, 2015a). There was no change in its structure, but a clear statement that councils represented the public interest, not that of professionals (PSA, 2013).

In 2014, the Law Commission, after close consultation with the professional councils, made recommendations for reform based on a broad consensus. If implemented, these will provide a new legal framework to simplify regulation. It will increase consistency and also allow greater flexibility to amend rules after agreement with the PSA. This cuts out the current clumsy and time-consuming process of seeking parliamentary approval for rule changes via section 60 of the NHS Reform and Health Professions Act 2002.

What has been the impact of the meta-regulator?

In the past, professional councils, their mode of governance and their policies were based on traditional practices and hidden from public view. The new forms of regulation have created new forms of knowledge. The councils are open to scrutiny and the public gaze through audit, accountability hearings and web-based publications. Transparency and accountability have increased and there are enhanced opportunities for dialogue. Through regular review, the meta-regulator has built an organisational memory. It can put pressure on the councils to identify and deal with problems and increase their efficiency. The PSA is able to influence, persuade and act as a conduit to the Department of Health. For example, following an audit of its FtP process, which was regarded as poorly managed with a huge backlog of cases, the NMC received an additional £20 million grant in 2012. This avoided raising the fees for registration, which was regarded as politically sensitive (DH, 2012).

The costs of introducing another layer of regulation have been considerable. Table 6.1 shows that the meta-regulator's income has more than doubled since 2003/04, from approximately £1.5 million to £3.4 million in 2014/15. The PSA now has indirect oversight of more registrants, professions and occupational groups. Since 2004/05, the number of FtP cases called in for review by the PSA has increased sevenfold from 590 in 2003/04 to 4,043 in 2014/15. From the evidence available in PSA annual reports (2015a, 2016a) the aim is to achieve greater consistency in processes and outcomes. Learning points from the reviews are passed back to the Councils. A small, but increased number of cases in each of these years were referred back to the High Court to consider whether the decision made had been 'unduly lenient' to the practitioner. Almost all related to decisions made by either the medical or nursing Council.

Since August 2015, the PSA's primary source of income is a levy on the regulatory bodies that it oversees. It will no longer be an arm's-length body of the Department of Health but a freestanding agency.

Table 6.1: Comparative data from the Council for Healthcare Regulatory Excellence 2003/04 and the Professional Standards Authority 2014/15

	Council for Healthcare Regulatory Excellence (CHRE) (2003/04)	Professional Standards Authority (PSA) (2014/15)
Number of registrants	1.1 million overseen by the nine professional councils	1.44 million overseen by the nine professional councils plus 65,000 practitioners on 18 accredited registers
Governing council Government appointments	19 members 9 regulators and 10 lay members	7 members representing the UK and the chief executive
Annual income – Department of Health	£1,450,000	£3,394,000
Staffing costs	£377,949	£1,982,000
Staff employed	10	35
Section 29 referrals*	**CHRE (2004/05)**	**PSA (2014/15)**
Number referred for review	590 reviewed	4,043 reviewed, 833 learning points fed back to regulators
Appeals to the High Court	8 referred	21 referred

Note: * Section 29 of the NHS Reform and Health Professions Act 2002.
Sources: CHRE and PSA annual reports

The professional councils: activity, diversity and barriers to change

Since the Health and Social Act 2008, each professional council board has been responsible for the strategic and operational oversight of its profession. It sets a framework for ensuring competence and behaviour and has, over the period, introduced its own reforms. We argue later in this chapter that regulatory activity within councils has increased, although we can only give illustrative examples here. Councils cannot oversee the day-to-day practice of many thousands of registrants. This is a shared responsibility with other regulators. As professionals, individuals are responsible for their own practice. In setting a framework for regulation, councils have a number of sources of intelligence. They can learn from complaints made by the public, from other regulators and stakeholders and from assessing the impact of changes in the broader social and economic environment. Some councils, notably the GMC and GDC, discuss in their annual reports how external factors shape their current regulatory strategy.

The increase in regulatory activity

Tables 6.2 and 6.3 show changes in the profile of each council and in selected areas of activity. We make a division between the smaller and larger councils for easier reading. Table 6.2 summarises the number of registrants, the number of staff members, income and registration fee of the smaller regulatory councils – the GCC, the GOC, the GOsC and the Pharmaceutical Society of Northern Ireland (PSNI) – in 2002/03 and in 2014/15, showing the changes between the two time points, unless where indicated. Even in this group, the diversity is remarkable. All four councils have an income of less than £10 million per annum. However, two councils (the GOC and PSNI) have seen a significant increase in income since 2002/03 – over 250%. Three of the four councils still have fewer than 5,000 registrants, although all have seen a rise in numbers. Most councils now employ more staff. In the GOC, staff levels have more than doubled, from 20 in 2005/06 to 49 in 2014/15. Registration fees remain the main source of income for all councils. Registration fees for the smaller councils are generally higher than those of the larger councils (summarised in Table 6.3). The costs of regulation are high, but the benefits of statutory regulation lead registrants to pay the fee.

Table 6.2: Smaller council registrants, staffing, income and annual registration fee, 2002/03 and 2014/15

	General Chiropractic Council (GCC)		General Optical Council (GOC)		General Osteopathic Council (GOsC)		Pharmaceutical Society Northern Ireland (PSNI)	
	2002/ 03	2014/ 15	2002/ 03	2014/ 15	2002/ 03	2014/ 15	2003/ 04	2014/ 15
Registrants (n)	2,019	3,034 (↑ 50%)	14,771	20,780* (↑ 41%)	3,225	4,975 (↑ 54%)	1,820	2,234* (↑ 23%)
Staff (n)	13	13.5	20**	49	21	28	N/A	13
Income (£ million)	1.912	2.372 (↑ 24%)	1.710	6.700 (↑ 292%)	2.308	2.771 (↑ 20%)	0.281	1.007 (↑ 258%)
Annual registration fee (£)	1,000	800	115	290	375– 750	320– 570	28–170	372

Notes: * Excludes premises. ** 2005/06 data.
Sources: Allsop et al (2004), councils' annual reports

The registrants, staffing, income and annual registration fee of the five larger councils – the GDC, GPhC, GMC, HCPC and NMC – are summarised in Table 6.3, which shows the relevant figures in the two time points 2002/03 and 2014/15, unless where indicated. Both the GDC and the HCPC had significant increases in registrants – 468% and 122% respectively. This was due to regulating additional groups. In 2004, the GDC register was expanded to include a range of specialist support staff; and in 2012, the HPC began to register social workers in England and was renamed the Health and Care Professions Council (HCPC). In all but the GPhC, both the number of staff and income increased between the two time points. In 2011, the GPhC register included pharmacy technicians although staff numbers and income fell. This may be due to a jurisdictional change as it regulates practising professionals only and not those in academia.

As corporate bodies, professional councils must balance their books and are subject to an annual financial audit. Income comes from fees and other sources. In 2014/15, the highest fees were paid by chiropractors and the lowest by nurses. This reflects their position in the labour market. Chiropractors are practitioners in the private sector while nurses are the largest group of professionals working within the NHS. Their level of pay is lower than, for example, doctors and dentists, so the level of the professional fee is politically sensitive and regulators have been reluctant to raise it. In 2014/15, the GCC and PSNI had the smallest number of staff and the smallest income, while the GMC had the largest budget and employed the largest number of staff of any council by far.

Regular checks on competence – revalidation and continuing professional development

The registration of professionals as competent to practise is a significant regulatory task particularly due to the increased mobility of health professionals. Most professional councils have streamlined their registration systems. According to the PSA (2015a), online methods have made registration a quicker, more straightforward and timely process and it has few criticisms about this activity. Public accessibility to registers has been enhanced, with more information on qualifications and specialisation. The registers also include information on restrictions on practice imposed in FtP hearings for five years.

Some factors that might be a risk to the public have been identified from cases investigated. We give two examples. In one instance, a panel hearing found that a doctor's practice was impaired due to poor language skills and, with pressure from the GMC, European Union regulations were renegotiated. Subsequently, a number of councils – the GDC, GPhC, NMC and PSNI, as well as the GMC – have introduced enhanced language testing for registration (Parkin, 2015). In a second instance, the GMC identified from its database a higher-than-expected incidence of complaints against doctors whose first qualification, then sufficient for registration, had been obtained overseas. Qualitative research found that junior doctors were often ill-prepared for practice in the UK and received poor support from their employers (Slowther et al, 2009). The identification of risk factors can enhance the protection of patients, although causal factors are not simple and must be unravelled. In terms of developing standards, the GMC is at the forefront of articulating the duties and responsibilities of professionals. Its booklet, *Good Medical Practice* (GMC, 2013), has been regarded best practice. Following the Inquiry into Mid Staffordshire NHS Foundation Trust by Francis (2013), its guidelines on whistleblowing and the duty of candour have been adopted by other councils.

The GMC has also taken a lead in annual licensing with periodic revalidation of competence every five years. Revalidation is based on a cumulative annual appraisal of competence based on a portfolio. The first round of revalidation ran from 2012 to 2016. Both employers and regulators must cooperate to ensure that the process is effective. The GMC liaises with employers to ensure that annual appraisals take place and have appointed regional officers to oversee the process (GMC, 2016). By 2016, the NMC had also commenced a revalidation programme (PSA, 2016a). Other councils have various forms of continuing professional development. In assessing these, the PSA

Table 6.3: Larger council registrants, staffing, income and annual registration fee, 2002/03 and 2014/15

	General Dental Council (GDC)		General Medical Council (GMC)		General Pharmaceutical Council (GPhC)		Health Professions Council (HPC) / Health and Care Professions Council (HCPC)		Nursing and Midwifery Council (NMC)	
	2002/03	2014/15	2002/03	2014/15	2002/03	2014/15	2003/04	2014/15	2002/03	2014/15
Registrants (n)	36,328	206,313 (↑ 468%)	203,398	267,169 (↑ 31%)	45,641	72,985* (↑ 60%)	149,242	330,887 (↑ 122%)	645,580	686,782 (↑ 6%)
Staff (n)	68	327 (↑ 381%)	340	945 (↑ 178%)	294	209 (↑ 29%)	60	215 (↑ 258%)	200	545 (↑ 173%)
Income (£ million)	4.661	33.140 (↑ 611%)	55.675	97.054 (↑ 74%)	26.308	20.475 (↑ 22%)	9.000**	26.303 (↑ 192%)	14.944	73.204 (↑ 389%)
Annual registration fee (£)	25/300	116/890	290	390	205***	108/240	60	80	20	120

Notes: * Excludes premises. ** 2004/05 data. *** 2004 figure.
Sources: Allsop et al (2004), council's annual reports

requires evidence that the programme is effective in protecting patients. Monitoring this is now a target for the PSA's next annual review.

Dealing with complaints

For all professional councils, the most challenging function is responding to concerns from the public about their registrants' FtP. The process is time-consuming and expensive. It is also the function where the public looks to the regulator to seek a response. Evidence suggests that the process is poorly understood and distressing for those who pursue a complaint. The GMC, following a pilot project to evaluate early meetings with people with a complaint, has appointed patient liaison officers based in Manchester to meet with complainants to explain the process. Meetings may take place before and after further investigation and final panel hearings (GMC, 2015). Additional support has also been provided for doctors (GMC, 2016).

Since 2002, the volume of cases that the professional councils process has increased at all stages, from the initial expressions of concern, to the cases investigated and panel hearings (see Tables 6.4 and 6.5). Numbers of suspensions and erasures from the register as an outcome from panel hearings have also increased over the period. The data must be treated with caution, as they are an indicator of activity only. Nevertheless, they suggest a growing administrative burden on councils. Table 6.4 shows the FtP data for the smaller councils. The GOsC had a 14% increase in the number of 'expressions of concern' between 2005/06 and 2014/15. In terms of timescales, in 2014/15 only one council (GOsC) took less than a year to deal with cases from receipt of the complaint to a final hearing – 51 weeks. The GCC took 72 weeks and the PSNI took 91 weeks. The GOC had the longest time from receipt of the complaint to a final hearing – 104 weeks (PSA, 2015a).

Table 6.5 shows the FtP data for the five larger professional councils. In all cases, the numbers of 'expressions of concern' have significantly increased. For some councils this growth may in part be due to the increase of professions or groups regulated. For example, the HCPC now registers more professions and includes social workers in England. Between 2003/04 and 2014/15, their expressions of concern rose in volume by 1,519% (over 16 times). The GDC, which now registers dental technicians, had a 240% increase between 2007 and 2014/15. Between 2003/04 and 2014/15, the NMC had a 280% increase, while the GMC and the GPhC had a 143% and 106% increase respectively. However, the number of expressions of concern still remains a very small percentage of registrants. By 2014/15, they ranged from less than

Table 6.4: Smaller council fitness to practise statistics, 2002/03 (or earliest available year) and 2014/15

	General Chiropractic Council (GCC)*		General Optical Council (GOC)		General Osteopathic Council (GOsC)		Pharmaceutical Society Northern Ireland (PSNI)*	
	2003/04	2014/15	2004/05	2014/15	2005/06	2014/15	2011/12	2014/15
Expressions of concern (n)	22	N/A	N/A	287	37	42	36	31
Referred for investigation (n)	11	N/A	182	279	N/A	42	N/A	N/A
Referred for FtP (n)	9	N/A	23	39	15	22	N/A	N/A
Suspensions or erasures (n)	N/A	4	9	12	2	5	N/A	2
Median time for receipt of complaint to final hearing	N/A	72 weeks	N/A	104 weeks	N/A	51 weeks	N/A	91 weeks

Notes: * Data for the GCC and PSNI were either incomplete or compiled over too short a time period to draw any conclusions. ** Figures given for cases referred for investigation/FtP and suspensions/erasures may include older cases that have carried forward.
Sources: Allsop et al (2004), PSA (2015a), councils' annual reports

1% for the HCPC, GOsC and NMC, less than 2% for the PSNI, GDC and GOC, to less than 3% of registrants for the GPhC and less than 4% for the GMC. For regulators dealing with cases, this is a significant, and costly, part of their work, although it provides an interface with the public as well as a source of intelligence.

The length of time taken to conclude cases is a matter of great concern to the PSA and no council has escaped criticism (PSA, 2015c). For 2014/15, the median for time taken for the five larger councils to process complaints from receipt of a complaint to a final hearing took over a year – the GDC took 93 weeks, the GMC 92, the GPhC 85, the NMC 81 and the HCPC 73. Many councils have made changes to their systems by introducing case managers, legally qualified or otherwise, with clear decision rules, and the PSA (2015c) has declared that all the regulators should be in a position to monitor case progression and make operational adjustments when delays occur.

In seven of the nine councils, the number of suspensions and erasures from the register has increased. Data are missing for the GCC and PSNI. This may reflect a backlog of cases from the past. The HCPC, NMC

Table 6.5: Larger council fitness to practise statistics, 2003/04 (or earliest available year) and 2014/15

	General Dental Council (GDC)		General Medical Council (GMC)		General Pharmaceutical Council (GPhC)		Health Professions Council (HPC) / Health and Care Professions Council (HCPC)		Nursing and Midwifery Council (NMC)	
	2007	2014/15	2003/04	2014/15	2011/12	2014/15	2003/04*	2014/15	2003/04	2014/15
Expressions of concern (n)	949	3,222 (↑240%)	3,962	9,637 (↑143%)	777	1,597 (↑106%)	134	2,170 (↑1,519%)	1,460	5,541 (↑280%)
Referred for investigation (n)	638	10,12	1,703	2,763	523	N/A	112	1,128	1,511	2,207
Referred for FtP (n)	118	403	79	237	N/A	N/A	45	849	283	971
Suspensions or erasures (n)	24	74 (↑208%)	140**	179 (↑28%)	55	89 (↑62%)	14	125 (↑793%)	186	874 (↑370%)
Median time for receipt of complaint to final hearing	N/A	93 weeks	N/A	92 weeks	N/A	85 weeks	N/A	73 weeks	N/A	81 weeks

Notes: * HPC – 112 allegations referred by screeners, 45 allegations referred by Investigating Committee Panel. ** Figure excludes 85 voluntary removals. * Figure given for cases referred for investigation/FtP and suspensions/erasures may include older cases that have carried forward.
Sources: Allsop et al (2004), PSA (2015a), councils' annual reports

and GDC saw significant rises (793%, 370% and 208% respectively). The increases for the GPhC (62%) and GMC (28%) were less, but the GMC has been on a rising trend for a decade until recently (Allsop and Jones, 2008).

Continuing diversity and the case for reform

Despite having a similar function and role, there remain substantial differences between the councils. These derive from their scale of operation, their position in the market and the constraints imposed on them by their founding legislation. This was a finding in our 2004 report for the CHRE (Allsop et al, 2004), and the differences, although reduced, remain, despite efforts by the meta-regulator to increase consistency. In 2014, the Law Commission (2014: 2) commented that professional regulation 'is neither systematic nor coherent and contains a wide range of inconsistencies and idiosyncrasies'. For example, the GPhC, GOC and PSNI license, register and inspect businesses and premises as well as individual practitioners. They can require businesses to employ particular professionals on their board of directors and may impose financial penalties for poor standards. Some councils, particularly those that cover professionals in private practice, still have a role in identifying and prosecuting people who are offering professional services without being registered.

Differences between councils are greatest in investigating complaints and disciplinary cases where terminology, process and powers still differ. For example, some regulators are introducing legally qualified FtP panel chairs as an alternative to using legal assessors and lay chairs. Others have a case examiner, who may be legally qualified with a range of powers:

- to conclude a case with no further action;
- to send a warning letter;
- to request a health or performance assessment;
- to make an interim application for suspension, pending further investigation.

The Law Commission (2014) recommended commonality in process and more flexibility to change rules. It proposed common procedures for registration, standards for practice and the investigation of allegations of impairment. Most importantly, it recommended a separation between the investigation of a complaint and its adjudication, an established legal principle.

The consultation by the Law Commission (2014) indicated a conflict of interest between the GMC and the PSA over the right to appeal decisions in disciplinary cases to the High Court. The GMC is currently able to appeal cases from its tribunal and wishes to maintain control, while the PSA considers this unnecessary as it has an appeal process, and considers that there is no added value in having two. The Law Commission concluded that both routes could stand. However, this issue may become part of the politics of reform in the next phase.

Most recently, the PSA (2016b) has suggested that the current draft Bill is insufficiently radical. It argues that the next Act governing the health professions must be both simple to understand and efficient, it suggests a split in the functions carried out by the councils and it argues that there should be a common register for all health and social care workers, as well as one agency to undertake investigations for the councils and one tribunal for the adjudication of cases. A consultation has been announced (Campbell, 2017).

The PSA also proposes the application of a model to assess risk for each profession and the use of a wider range of options for dealing with some complaints. Its perspective is that of a corporate rationaliser and justified in terms of efficiency and simplicity. If taken forward, these proposals would have major implications. The proposal to split functions is likely to be resisted as it would change the ability of councils to control the range of functions for their profession. Professional regulators rely on their registrants internalising norms of practice as they are accountable for their own decisions. The proposals might fracture the notion of belonging to a community and a sense of a collective identity.

Conclusion

The reforms in the regulation of health and social care professionals now aim to protect users of their expert services from harm. Professional regulators can only do this at one remove by:

- setting standards for practice in education and training;
- registering those who are competent by virtue of qualification;
- overseeing the reassessment of competence through revalidation;
- responding to expressions of concern through investigation;
- adjudicating a case where a registrant may be deemed not fit to practise;
- suspending or removing a registrant from the register – the final sanction.

These functions have long been in place but, over time, professional regulation has been extended to more groups, with minor adjustments. Since 2002, what has changed?

The first change is structural. The meta-regulator, the PSA, is distanced from government and particular interests. It sets a policy steer for good practice in regulation. It has a developed a comprehensive set of standards against which to assess councils' performance through review and audit. From the available evidence, and despite a lack of powers for enforcement, it appears that there has been a shift towards greater consistency in regulatory practice through the collaborative effort of councils and the meta-regulator. The PSA continues to investigate how professional and accredited regulators might identify risks to the public in their area of practice. This requires further development but some regulators have identified what could be risk factors and, in consequence, made changes. In this chapter we have also pointed to structural changes in professional councils. These councils now maintain a distance from professional interests. The focus of the council in setting strategy and managing regulatory functions in the public interest lies with an enlarged executive with, as we have shown, a growth in the administrative function.

A second change has been the influence of the legal gaze following inquiries. As expressions of concern have risen, the management of FtP processes has become a major focus in most councils. The process of the investigation of cases is now shaped by decision rules, and administrative and external legal input, and is separated from adjudication. In some of the larger councils, this is manifest by a physical separation of functions. The PSA provides an additional layer of scrutiny over an increasing volume of cases, with powers to refer to the High Court in the interest of equity and fairness. Again, a distancing of the regulator from professional interests is evident.

A third change has been an increase in transparency and accountability. Before the reform process began, professional regulation took place behind closed doors and was a neglected area of public policy. Both the meta-regulator and the professional councils are now more open to scrutiny in terms of reporting and both are accountable to the Health Committee. There are new sources of knowledge. Compared with the past, there is more information about the policies and practice of regulators on the web and in print media. Of course, there are limits to openness. The administrative decisions within the councils in the investigation of cases are rule-bound but opaque. The anonymity of the parties is protected in a dispute prior to the panel or tribunal hearing, which is in public.

Professional councils are more fit for purpose than in the past, but challenges remain. Those who use services often have a poor understanding of what to expect from professionals and of the role of regulators. For regulators, further legislation is necessary to increase flexibility in processes and so is close collaboration between employers and regulators to share information that could prevent harm. As a consequence of the increase in regulatory activity, the costs of regulation have risen. There are also questions about the capacity of councils to meet the higher standards expected: are some too small and others too large? Two certainties are that the reform process will continue and, as far as patients are concerned, professionalism and adherence to good standards are as necessary as ever. A major challenge is to maintain a balance in regulation between professional autonomy and external surveillance.

References

Allsop, J. and Jones, K. (2008) 'Citizens or consumers: complaints in healthcare settings', *Social Policy and Society* 7(2): 233–43.

Allsop, J., Jones, K., Meerabeau, L., Mulcahy, L. and Price, D. (2004) *Regulating the Health Professions – A Scoping Exercise*, London: Council for the Regulation of the Healthcare Professions.

Better Regulation Task Force (2003) *Principles of Good Regulation*, London: Better Regulation Task Force.

Campbell, D. (2017) 'Jeremy Hunt to consider merging health regulation bodies', *The Guardian*, 8 February, https://www.theguardian.com/politics/2017/feb/08/jeremy-hunt-to-consider-merging-health-regulation-bodies

CHRE (Council for Healthcare Regulatory Excellence) (2004) *Annual Report 2003/4*, London: CHRE.

CHRE (2012) *Performance Review Report 2011/12*, London: CHRE.

Day, P. and Klein, R. (1997) *Steering But Not Rowing: Transformation of the Department of Health*, Bristol: Policy Press.

de Bere, S. R., Bryce, M., Archer, J., Nunn, S., Lynn, N. and Roberts, M. (2014) *Review of Decision-Making in the General Medical Council's Fitness to Practise Procedures*, Plymouth: University of Plymouth.

DH (Department of Health) (2006a) *Good Doctors, Safer Patients: Proposals to Strengthen the System to Assure and Improve the Performance of Doctors and to Protect the Safety of Patients*, London: DH.

DH (2006b) *The Regulation of the Non-Medical Healthcare Professions*, London: DH.

DH (2007a) *Safeguarding Patients: The Government's Response to the Recommendations of the Shipman Inquiry's Fifth Report and to the recommendations of the Ayling, Neale and Kerr/Haslam Inquiries*, Cm 7015, London: DH.

DH (2007b) *Trust, Assurance and Safety: The Regulation of Health Professionals*, London: DH.

DH (2011) *Enabling Excellence: Autonomy and Accountability for Health and Social Care Staff*, Cm 8008, London: DH.

DH (2012) 'Government offers £20 million grant to the Nursing and Midwifery Council', press release, 15 October, London: DH.

Donaldson, L. (2000) *Organisation with a Memory: Learning from Adverse Events in the NHS*, London: Department of Health.

Felstiner, W., Abel, R. and Sarat, A. (1981) 'The emergence and transformation of disputes', *Law and Society Review* 15: 631-54.

Fenton, L. and Salter, B. (2009) 'Competition and compromise in negotiating the new governance of medical performance', *Health, Economics, Policy and Law* 4: 283-303.

Flynn, N. (2012) *Public Sector Management* (6th edition), London: Sage.

Francis, R. (2013) *Report of the Mid Staffordshire NHS Foundation Trust Public Inquiry*, London: The Stationery Office.

GDC (General Dental Council) (2014) *Annual Report and Accounts 2013/14*, London: GDC.

GMC (General Medical Council) (2000) *Proposals for Revalidation*, Manchester: GMC.

GMC (2013) *Good Medical Practice*, Manchester: GMC.

GMC (2015) *Patient Liaison Service*, Manchester: GMC.

GMC (2016) *Working for Patients, Working with Doctors: Annual Report 2015/16*, Manchester: GMC.

Hood, C., Rothstein, H. and Baldwin, R. (2001) *The Government of Risk: Understanding Risk Regulation Regimes*, New York, NY: Oxford University Press.

House of Lords (2016) *Regulation of Health and Social Care Professions in England*, HL Bill 24, London: The Stationery Office.

Hutter, B. M. (2005) *The Attractions of Risk-Based Regulation: Accounting for the Emergence of Risk Ideas in Regulation*, CARR paper 33, London: London School of Economics.

Irvine, D. (2003) *The Doctors' Tale: Professionalism and Public Trust*, Oxford: Radcliffe Medical Press.

Kagan, R. A. (1989) 'Understanding regulatory enforcement: editor's introduction', *Law and Policy* 2(2): 89-119.

Kirkup, B. (2015) *The Report of the Morecambe Bay Investigation*, London: The Stationery Office.

Law Commission (2014) *Regulation of Health Care Professionals: Regulation of Social Care Professionals in England*, Cm 8839, London: The Stationery Office.

Lloyd-Bostock, S. and Hutter, B. H. (2008) 'Reforming regulation in the medical profession: the risks of risk-based approaches', *Health Risk and Society* 10(1): 69-83.

Parkin, E. (2015) *Language Testing for Healthcare Professionals*, briefing paper 07267, London: House of Commons Library.

Pharmaceutical Journal (2010) 'Adjudication of fitness-to-practise cases may no longer be taken over by independent organisation', *Pharmaceutical Journal*, 11 August, www.pharmaceutical-journal.com/news-and-analysis/news/adjudication-of-fitness-to-practise-cases-may-no-longer-be-taken-over-by-independent-organisation/11020779.article

PSA (Professional Standards Authority) (2013) *Fit and Proper? Governance in the Public Interest*, London: PSA.

PSA (2015a) *Annual Report 2014/2015*, London: PSA.

PSA (2015b) *Right-Touch Regulation: Revised*, London: PSA.

PSA (2015c) *Annual Report: Accounts and Performance Review 2014/15 Volume II Performance Report 2014/15*, London: PSA, www.professionalstandards.org.uk/publications/performance-review-detail/performance-review-2014-2015

PSA (2016a) *Annual Report 2015/2016*, London: PSA.

PSA (2016b) *Regulation Rethought*, London: PSA.

Saks, M. and Allsop, J. (2007) 'Social policy, professional regulation and health support work in the UK', *Social Policy and Society* 6(2): 165-77.

Salter, B. (2007) 'Governing UK medical performance: a struggle for policy dominance', *Health Policy* 8(23): 263-75.

Slowther, A., Hundt, G., Taylor, R. and Purkis, J. (2009) *Non-UK Qualified Doctors and Good Medical Practice: Report*, London: General Medical Council.

Smith, J. (2004) *The Shipman Inquiry: Fifth Report: Safeguarding Patients: Lessons from the Past – Proposals for the Future*, Cm 6394, London: The Stationery Office.

SEVEN

Regulation and Russian medicine: whither medical professionalisation?

Mike Saks

Introduction

Globally, the regulation of medicine has been a high priority for governments (see, for instance, Kuhlmann and Saks, 2008). Classically in the modern developed world – and especially in the Anglo-American context – this has taken the form in occupational terms from a neo-Weberian perspective of exclusionary social closure, legally sanctioned by the state (Saks, 2016). Although this has been subject to dilution in some countries with growing corporatisation and concern about the protection offered to citizens, the general template of social closure in the field of medicine has involved the creation of self-regulated professional monopolies in the market (Saks, 2015). Russia, however, stands out as a society that has never had a fully autonomously regulated profession of medicine in this sense, with state-sanctioned insiders and outsiders, independent self-control of practitioners and all the income, status and power with which this is typically associated. As such, it is an interesting international case from the viewpoint of professional health regulation in the public interest, especially given the frequent current association of professions in general and the medical profession in particular in neo-Weberian work with the pursuit of self-interests at the expense of the overall welfare (see, among others, Saks, 1995). This is not to say, of course, that there are no regulatory controls over physicians, nor that there have not been shifts in the nature of these over time. Indeed, this chapter seeks to chart both these controls and the changes in these historically and contemporaneously – including through the tumultuous impact of the Russian Revolution on the incipient medical profession and the founding of the Soviet Union in the early 20th century.

Medical regulation in early modern times

At the start of the early modern period from the 17th century onwards in the vast expanse of Russia, the country was characterised by the more or less unfettered operation of traditional practitioners of folk medicine such as herbalism and bone setting competing in a relatively open market – much like the parallel position in countries such as Britain and the United States (US) (Porter, 2002). Such practitioners did not typically have university education and their craft was self-taught or based on apprenticeships. Physicians, however, gradually began to be drawn from abroad to minister to members of the court and nobility. This presaged their growing role as functionaries of the state, which increased further with the needs of the expanding military in Imperial Russia (Field, 1967). At this point, though, the work of the small number of university-educated, high-status and well-rewarded doctors was not yet based on a systematic theoretical body of thought. Nonetheless they were employed on a patronage basis to provide services for the highest echelons of society, including the Tsar, in a distinctive system of state engagement that led to the development of indigenous hospital medical schools in the latter part of the 17th century. In terms of regulation, control over student entry and examinations for these schools were shared between the state and physicians, although doctors had more independence over clinical decision making (Frieden, 1981).

Both the indigenous and better-rewarded overseas doctors, however, were overseen by the Apothecary Board, which developed into the Medical Collegium towards the end of the 18th century. Significantly, as Field (1967) relates, this regulatory institution was subordinated to the Tsar's family and had jurisdiction over hospitals, pharmacists and doctors. A Medical Registration Act was also passed in Russia in the early 18th century setting up a licensing system for those physicians with accredited qualifications who were deemed competent to practise, with legal protection of the title of 'doctor'. Although this could be seen as an early form of exclusionary closure, there was only limited self-regulation as physicians continued to come under the sway of the state – in which the standing of medical officials was generally greater than medical practitioners, especially those of Russian extraction (Frieden, 1981). Indeed, given the short supply of medical practitioners at the time, the state imposed severe criminal penalties on doctors if they left their positions to follow other careers or did not respond to official calls for action (Yurchenko, 2004). While the numbers of doctors increased with the ever-growing spread and standardisation of higher-level medical education, by the mid-19th century a distinctive, potentially competing, group of *feldshers* with a shorter training to cope with the excess demand had emerged and the Medical Collegium had been replaced by the Medical Department of the Ministry of Internal Affairs, which remained in control of medicine in a largely uncoordinated health system (Field, 1967).

The position of doctors, though, can be seen as 'professionalisation from above' in an ever-more pluralistic health field in which a small number of elite university-trained physicians with rich clients in big cities operated alongside *feldshers* and a broader range of lower-status folk practitioners ministering to the wider population in a predominantly agricultural society (Yurchenko, 2004). But this changed with moves towards a more Anglo-American model of 'professionalisation from within' (McClelland, 1991) following the emancipation of the serfs in 1861 in Russia, which led to the development of *zemstvos*, a form of district local government (Hosking, 2012). This system provided free medical care involving doctors and *feldshers* beyond simply the urban middle and upper classes. Although they were not generally well paid, *zemstvo* physicians had greater independence outside the patronage of high-paying clients and the Tsarist state. This was reflected in their growing conflict with district managers, in a battle for regulatory autonomy as opposed to autocracy, and with *feldshers* and folk practitioners who increasingly became direct competitors (Hyde, 1974). Nonetheless, with a growing sense of identity, fuelled in part by their ever-stronger commitment to biomedicine, doctors were able to form various professionalising medical organisations – not least in 1881 the nationally based Pirogov Society, which lobbied for medical, social and political reform (Frieden, 1981).

The main aims of the Pirogov Society included increasing solidarity among doctors, expanding their prestige and independence to parallel medicine in Western societies and maintaining control of the workplace (Schecter, 1997). However, Tsarist opposition to self-regulation meant that officials in the powerful Ministry of Internal Affairs blocked attempts to establish a Ministry of Health outside the medical bureaucracy (Solomon and Hutchinson, 1990). From this point onwards, members of the Pirogov Society increasingly realised that its efforts to enhance the socio-political position of doctors were inextricably linked to transcending the Tsarist regime. From 1904, therefore, doctors began to organise into unions to represent their views, including first the All-Russian Union of Medical Personnel and then the All-Russian Union of Professional Associations of Physicians (Field, 1967). In February 1917, Tsarism was eventually overthrown and a provisional government was formed. In the months that followed, the Pirogov Society was permitted to lead medical professional reform, with the new Central Medical-Sanitary Council organising medical services in liaison with government (Yurchenko, 2004). This quickly resulted in an independent health service run by doctors and financed by local insurance and private funding (Navarro, 1977), with a medical profession with shared values and a relatively autonomous role in directing medicine – including oversight of entry to medical schools and the content of medical examinations (Field, 1967). Although their status was limited, male and increasing numbers of female doctors had at last come within touching distance of establishing a self-regulatory profession based on exclusionary social closure underwritten by the state. However, the medical regulatory landscape shifted fundamentally after the Bolshevik Revolution of October 1917.

The deprofessionalisation of medicine following the 1917 Russian Revolution

When the Bolsheviks displaced the provisional government in October 1917, Lenin sought to establish a socialist regime with land acquisition by the peasantry, workers' control in the factories and a one-party rule in the transition from capitalism to communism (Service, 2009). After the Civil War of 1918 to 1921, therefore, the Soviet Union was established, comprised of Russia and other member states of its previous Empire. A short period of War Communism followed marked by the nationalisation of private property, after which the New Economic Policy was introduced later in the 1920s to revitalise the economy by reintroducing the private market on a selective basis (Hosking, 2012). In this highly politicised environment, the consequence of Communist Party control for the regulation of doctors remained extreme and was not helped by the fact that the Pirogov Society had opposed the regime in fear of being reduced to proletarian standing, calling on doctors to sabotage health care (Navarro, 1977). Given the massive public health difficulties facing Russia both during and after the Civil War – not least typhus, cholera and famine (Tulchinsky and Varavikova, 2014) – it is not surprising that the Bolsheviks tended to see physicians from the old regime as class enemies. Accordingly, at a national level they replaced the Central Medical-Sanitary Council with the Central People's Commissariat of Health and gave responsibility for health locally to Soviets, comprised of elected peasants and industrial workers, which employed physicians working outside the private market on a salaried basis (Yurchenko, 2004).

In turn, the Bolsheviks also undermined the All-Russian Union of Professional Associations of Physicians by supporting the pro-regime All-Russian Union of Medical Workers initially comprised primarily of *feldshers* and later by groups such as pharmacists and nurses (Hyde, 1974). After the Communist Party dissolved the Union of Professional Associations of Physicians, doctors in public practice were allowed to affiliate with the Union of Medical Workers, which was a requirement for state employment and organised around broad fields of application, as opposed to the specialisms of the Pirogov Society (Navarro, 1977). Crucially, following the formal disestablishment of the Pirogov Society in 1925 and the reform of the organisation of medical care, any substantial lingering elements of medical regulatory independence disappeared, along with the identification of physicians as a socio-political elite (Schecter, 1997). Consequently, some neo-Weberian commentators have talked of the 'deprofessionalisation' of medicine under state socialism in the Soviet Union (see, for instance, Yurchenko, 2004). However, under socialism, the stronger Marxist concept of 'proletarianisation' may be more appropriate to describe the diminishing position of doctors in this period (McKinlay and Arches, 1985). Field (1957: 45) sees this transformation as turning 'a self-conscious, independent, vocal, politically oriented, and militant corporate entity' into 'a docile and politically inert employee group', in which the Soviet regime called the shots.

Admittedly, Brown (1987) has contested such claims, arguing, among other things, that they exaggerate the autonomous standing of Russian physicians before the Russian Revolution and their oppositional stance towards the Bolsheviks. But her position is weakened by the highly selective group of psychiatric doctors on which she bases her account – as they were known to be especially critical of Tsarism and favourably disposed towards democracy and egalitarianism (Sirotkina, 2010). Moreover, it is beyond dispute that, by the time of the Stalinist period from the late 1920s onwards, the medical spontaneity and discretion permitted under the provisional government had been replaced by extensive Communist Party-led bureaucratic regulatory constraints in the Soviet Union (Field, 1957). This was facilitated by a threefold growth in the numbers of Soviet physicians driven by the Party between 1917 and 1928, largely through the increasing recruitment to medical schools of women, peasants and industrial workers, which undermined the economic market position of doctors (Navarro, 1997). This was exacerbated by a further tenfold expansion from the 1920s of doctors, engineers and scientists in the subsequent years of the Soviet Union – the highest increase in the modern industrial world (Yurchenko, 2004).

Although doctors retained some of the traditional status of intellectuals, this also contributed to the emaciation of medical power in a system dominated by the Communist Party (Mansurov et al, 2004).

In this respect, the Marxist–Leninist philosophy on which the Soviet Union was in name established, castigated capitalist health systems and sought a revolutionary change in medicine under socialism in which classes spawned by private property were to be abolished. This resulted in Soviet medicine espousing the ensuing main principles from its inception:

- health care was a responsibility and function of the state;
- its development needed to occur within a single plan;
- health services should be administratively and bureaucratically centralised;
- health and related services must be accessible to the population without direct cost;
- prevention more than clinical intervention should be at the heart of the medical system;
- medical theory and practice should be brought together founded on research;
- medical care should be supported by the public wherever feasible;
- prioritisation is necessary given that medical services are a scarce resource (Field, 2000).

In addition, these principles were complemented by a commitment to achieving greater equality between groups – with particular reference to industrial workers as a key factor in a socialist system. Within this tightly centralised egalitarian framework, in contrast to such capitalist societies as Britain and the US, by the end of the 1920s Soviet doctors were generally paid at a lower rate than manual industrial labourers, lacked self-regulated autonomy, and had lost much of their significance in the political pecking order (Allsop et al, 1999). What, then, were the more detailed regulatory consequences for medicine of Stalin's leadership up to the early 1950s and his successors thereafter as the Soviet Union developed?

Medical regulation in the subsequent years of the Soviet Union

Here it must be said that Stalin led a regime that, unlike its liberal democratic counterparts, appeared totalitarian as well as authoritarian – with power focused in a leader with a wide span of control over key functions such as the armed forces, the economy, mass media and the police (Geyer and Fitzpatrick, 2009). This allowed him to conduct periodic mass purges to suppress opposition inside and outside the Communist Party, in which millions were executed or sent to labour camps (Hosking, 2012). This concentration of power also enabled Stalin ruthlessly to effect modernisation through five-year plans aimed at rapid industrialisation and the mechanisation and collectivisation of agriculture, in an increasingly politically isolated society in which he came to emphasise the benefits of 'socialism in one country' (Service, 2009). This did not bode well for the regulation of medicine, which was seen as a potentially subversive area, while at the same time being a central instrument in maintaining the working and fighting capacity of the Soviet Union. As such, from the outset, the Health Commissariat and later its successor, the Ministry of Health, were directed by the Central Committee of the Communist Party to address public health issues arising from urbanisation and agrarian reform, with prioritisation given to industrial workers (Navarro, 1977). This meant:

- following Communist Party dictates in supporting preventive over clinical services;
- dividing medical schools into faculties of general medicine, paediatrics and public health;
- introducing polyclinics to supply district-level primary care, from which the hospital-affiliated specialists employed could make referrals (Fry, 2012).

The polyclinic in turn was linked to teams of doctors working at micro-district level and situated in a centralised hierarchical structure, with the Republican Ministries of Health at its apex. This system helped to mitigate the huge human costs associated with the engagement of the Soviet Union in the Second World War, based as it was on a limited territorial/residential network for the general population and a superior closed/departmental network for those in higher occupations/ranks such as the political elite (Field, 2000). However, it had its frailties from a socialist perspective – not least that the principle of free access was not always in evidence due, among other things, to the fees charged for more qualified medical practitioners and reducing waiting times, the existence of a black market in medicine, and the continuing availability of private practice (Ryan, 1989). Substantively, though, the ever-escalating rate of production of doctors in the absence of an autonomously regulated medical profession meant that there were twice the proportion of doctors to population relative to Britain and the US (Field, 1967).

Physicians in this framework possessed six-year higher education credentials followed by internships, albeit with lower entry standards to medical schools and a more broadly based social intake than in pre-revolutionary times (Read, 1990). There was also a strong preponderance of women, which – aside from emancipatory socialist policy – could be seen to symbolise the decline in the position of medicine (Harden, 2001). This is despite growing medical specialisation in gynaecology and paediatrics and the importance of expert physicians in developing norms and standards, in association with the Minister of Health who was always drawn from medical ranks (Navarro, 1977). The reduced standing of doctors in the Stalinist period was underlined by the ongoing absence of exclusionary closure and the more egalitarian structure of the Union of Medical Workers, reflected in the lower-grade tasks normally performed by *feldshers* and nurses that they undertook in heavily doctored areas (Field, 1967). Indeed, the latter staff often had authority over old-style bourgeois physicians in decision making, especially if they were Communist Party members (Field, 2000). Against this, doctors retained their provenance over the fringe area of complementary and alternative medicine, given strong state support for using scientific biomedicine to serve the masses, resulting in the formalised marginality of folk practitioners (Yurchenko and Saks, 2006).

When Stalin died in 1953, Khrushchev denounced him and the excesses of the repression purges became less apparent (Service, 2009). After the fall of Khrushchev in the early 1960s, a succession of leaders took over, including Brezhnev and his acolytes Andropov and Chernenko. Gorbachev then came to power in the mid-1980s when liberal reforms were introduced to ensure more democratisation based on *glasnost* relating to openness and *perestroika*, presaging the restructuring that was to occur (Sakwa, 2010). This led to the dissolution of the Soviet Union in 1991 after a period of shortages, budget deficits, inflationary increases and secession by some constituent states. However, the years leading up to this maintained considerable consistency with the past as far as the regulation of doctors in Russia was concerned. Having said this, there were some shifts – not least from the limited decentralisation of the Khrushchev era to the more centralised Communist Party-based approach under Brezhnev (Hosking, 2012). Brezhnev ensured that primary care was even more firmly positioned at the base of a bureaucratic hierarchy bounded by secondary care and highly specialised tertiary care, followed by regional and republican layers under the Ministry of Health and reporting to the Council of

Ministers – alongside the regional and national research institutes and the high-status Russian Academy of Medical Sciences (Navarro, 1977).

In this system of medical care, which continued to be marked by corruption (Bernstein et al, 2010) – in tandem with many incompetent physicians, unsuitable hospital buildings and limited supplies of equipment and pharmaceuticals (Field, 2000) – polyclinics remained the main delivery system for primary care, with an ever-more specialised medical labour force in the increasingly important hospital sector (Fry, 2012). Legislation enacted in the late 1940s and 1950s enhanced the continuity of patient care (Navarro, 1977), but the top-down bureaucratic central planning and coordination remained – tempered by moves in the last years of the Soviet regime to greater privatisation (Yurchenko, 2004). This was designed to offset the growing shortage of public resources devoted to health care (Davis, 1989), paralleled by the desire to maintain a state-supported two-tiered medical system with preferential treatment for industrial workers and the Communist Party elite (Field, 2000). To be sure, some individual doctors managed to avoid being posted on the basis of need to less attractive rural areas where cultural and working conditions were generally inferior, but in general terms their highly state-regulated position, with lower-than-national average salaries, was maintained – not aided in terms of market positioning by the fact that by the 1960s one quarter of medical staff worldwide were Soviet physicians (Field, 1967).

Even if the Communist Party was still the main arbiter of medical decision making – including the notorious use of psychiatry against political dissidents through the KGB from the 1960s to the 1980s (Savelli and Marks, 2015) – doctors retained an element of control over clinical performance, medical education and disciplinary procedures, as well as their increasingly popular competitors in complementary and alternative medicine operating primarily in the private fee-for-service and self-help sectors (Yurchenko, 2004). However, the general deprofessionalisation of physicians in the post-Stalin era was accentuated by ongoing majority female representation in the medical workforce, the relatively large proportion of paramedical tasks undertaken by doctors and the greater autonomy given to ancillary groups, particularly in allied health and *feldsher* stations in the countryside (Field, 2000). This, though, started to be reversed through a process of reprofessionalisation of medicine following the transition from Soviet to post-Soviet times in the early 1990s (Coulter et al, 2006) – in which first the Confederation of Independent States and then the Russian Federation superseded the Soviet Union (Henderson, 2011). It is to this transition and its regulatory implications for physicians, with greater emphasis on the private market and democratic process as opposed to a monolithic one-party state, which the analysis now turns.

The reprofessionalisation of medicine in Russia in the post-Soviet era

The Russian Federation was created in 1991 when Yeltsin became President following the dissolution of the Soviet Union and its planned economy. This led to liberalising reforms, during which the Gross Domestic Product and industrial output initially fell substantially as private individuals took control of state enterprises (Service, 2009). This was associated with increases in crime and corruption in Russia, growing conflicts with indigenous minority populations, rising levels of poverty and escalating death rates (Field and Twigg, 2000). These trends were attenuated under Putin who took on the presidency in 2000, after a brief period as Prime Minister. When Medvedev became President in 2008, Putin went back to being Prime Minister until 2012, after which they switched roles. In this period, Putin brought greater stability and economic growth, despite his increasingly authoritarian and parochial nationalistic approach that had more in common with the Soviet Union than Western democracy (Sakwa, 2014). Nonetheless, with the removal of the Communist Party and market reform, the doors were opened to potential regulatory change and the reprofessionalisation of medicine, although this was not on the immediate agenda because of the chaos caused by the transition from one political system to another.

Indeed, the successive economic crises linked to the rapid dismantling of the Soviet Union at first prompted reductions in health funding, which contributed to the widespread epidemics in Russia in the 1990s (Davidova et al, 2009). The associated falls in life expectancy were also exacerbated by the significant regional variability in health provision, with the market-incentivised devolution that followed – as enterprises assigned too little income to this area in a confusing blend of state and private engagement in medical care (Twigg, 2001). As a report by the Organisation for Economic Co-operation and Development (OECD, 2012) on the health system under the Russian Federation indicates, at a time of rising medical costs, shortfalls in the funding landscape seriously and detrimentally affected the quality of medicine, as well as inequalities of access related to geographical, financial and other factors. Against this, though, the report notes that public funding of free health service entitlement has since increased within the framework of the Mandatory Health Insurance system and the Government Guarantee

Package, assisted by the National Priority Programme providing emergency health funding – even if more attention needs to be given to areas such as the coordination, continuity, cost-effectiveness and efficiency of medical care, along with payment systems, prevention and primary care. Oversight of state and private medical institutions by the Federal Service for Supervision of Consumer Protection and Human Welfare and the Federal Service on Surveillance in Healthcare and Social Development, though, promises further advances.

For all the changes, however, legacy issues have heavily impacted on the new system. For example, in a study at the turn of the 21st century on the new Russia, while doctors had greater freedom to move from state to private practice to enhance their earnings, they generally did not do so as a result of their attachment to socialised medicine – underpinned by their desire for a low-cost service for disadvantaged people, especially for life-threatening conditions and immediate wellbeing (Mansurov and Yurchenko, 2011). In a similar vein, most doctors in this study only wanted limited privatisation of the medical market in line with the views of the general public (Twigg, 2002), alongside the continuance of the Soviet practice of 'under-the-counter' payments in cash or kind (Nazarova, 2009). Moreover, although the heads of medical institutions wished to improve clinical standards and performance, physicians on the ground felt that there was insufficient local discretion in a system where medical prices and pay in self-financing areas were determined centrally, along with medical appointments (Yurchenko, 2004). This is indicative of the legacy of the lack of professional self-regulation, as the Ministry of Health has not allowed doctors or other allied health groups to govern themselves (Moskovskaya et al, 2013).

In this light, it is not surprising that physicians do not currently normally turn to medical associations for support as they are seen as ineffective given the continuing power of state bureaucracy (Yurchenko, 2004). This is indicated by the fact that most doctors suffered a fall in income in the Russian Federation, which has led to extended working hours and a still-heavier dependence on informal gifts from patients (Allsop et al, 1999). Having said this, despite more fragmentary working arrangements, medical practitioners still have a common identity based on their expertise and altruistic ideology (Mansurov and Yurchenko, 2011). Moreover, although doctors lack experience of self-regulation (Field, 2000), there is increasing interest more generally in establishing professional associations based on scientific knowledge (Geltzer, 2009). Indeed, a number of these have emerged in medicine and other occupations, but none yet seem capable of regulating practitioners across the entire Russian Federation (Moskovskaya et al, 2013) – even if in medicine they have developed a track record of organising scholarly discussions in various forums, including seminars and conferences (Prisyazhnyuk and Sadykov, 2012). Nonetheless, more politically oriented, interest-based medical practitioner organisations have now begun to emerge in the new Russia (Yurchenko, 2004).

This is illustrated by the Russian Medical Association, which primarily comprises public sector doctors. This body has been less than comfortable with the state reducing physician involvement in health care and the inadequate levels of funding for the new health insurance scheme. Drawing on symbolic references to the Pirogov Society, it has aimed to strengthen its position through the state, while enhancing the standing and pay of medical practitioners, as well as their place in decision making, through 'professionalisation from above'. Accordingly, it has expressed its desire for its members to be more involved federally and locally in the Fund for Compulsory Health Insurance to establish a legal framework for physicians – setting out professional standards, terms of reference for licensing and accreditation arrangements (Mansurov and Yurchenko, 2011). Its aspirational competitor body, the Russian Association of Private Medical Practitioners, with a stronger private sector constituency, has in contrast sought to advance the cause of an independent medical profession with a legal monopoly, a single register, and central engagement in accreditation, licensing and pricing in the medical market. Its strategic regulatory aim from a neo-Weberian perspective more closely follows the Anglo-American model of medical self-regulation, based on 'professionalisation from within' (Yurchenko, 2004). As such, it could be viewed as a potential instrument for classic reprofessionalisation in the Russian Federation, paralleling and building on the position reached under the provisional government immediately before the Russian Revolution (Frieden, 1981).

However, following Tsarism in Imperial Russia, the state has not wished to cede power (Moskovskaya et al, 2013), This has resulted in doctors and their associations – which are distanced from the lives and labour of medical practitioners on the ground – still only having comparatively weak control of medical entry, licensing, medical examinations, medical workforce numbers, poorly performing doctors and codes of ethics (Yurchenko, 2004). This is underlined by the relatively low financial rewards of Russian physicians internationally (Tulchinsky and Varavikova, 2014), even though average medical income is higher than it was at the outset of the New Russia, notwithstanding ongoing gender divisions (Harden, 2001). It is paradoxical that self-regulation has been more fully realised by the owners of hospitals and polyclinics than physicians, despite inconsistent regional accreditation and quality standards (OECD, 2012). Against this, doctors have largely held off the challenge by both other orthodox health practitioners and unorthodox therapists. The case of the latter, ranging from naturopaths to psychic healers, is particularly interesting given the popular countercultural resurgence in Russia over the past two or three decades linked to mainstream health shortfalls (Iarskaia-Smirnova and Romanov, 2008). Medical dominance has been maintained here with the support of the Ministry of Health; it has encouraged state physicians to incorporate more biomedically based aspects of complementary medicine such as acupuncture and osteopathy by legally restricting their use to physicians and offering education and training for doctors in such areas (Yurchenko and Saks, 2006). The main exception due to public pressure has been the selective licensing of indigenous folk healers (Salo, 2009) and the legalisation of the medical practice of homeopathy, although this remains a marginal specialty (Prisyazhnyuk and Sadykov, 2012).

Conclusion

The continuance of state control in the regulation of doctors is highlighted by the State Nomenclature of Doctors and Pharmacists' Specialties, as inclusion on this list gives rights to use public consulting rooms and to provide medical care free of charge on medical referral (Yurchenko, 2004). This represents a form of social closure, as also indicated by state-led restrictions on the disbursement of research funding and the content of the medical curriculum. However, it is not the type of self-regulatory exclusionary closure that has underpinned medical professionalisation in modern Western societies, especially in the Anglo–American context. This is underlined by the fact that doctors only serve as advisers on state accreditation boards that register doctors (Yurchenko and Saks, 2006). Accordingly, there are real limits on the extent to which physicians can be said to have reprofessionalised in the current ever-more directly managed market under Putin, in which state-owned companies constitute the majority of the economy and state and private insurance foundations are growing in control (Sakwa, 2014). To be sure, the life expectancy of the population is again increasing with more consistent medical accreditation and growing funding of the more technologically sophisticated health system through taxation, social contributions and direct payments – despite ongoing issues related to insurance coverage, the quality of pharmaceutical provision, access to medical care and the strategic leadership of health services (OECD, 2012). However, the prospects for medical professionalisation in neo-Weberian terms remain in the balance moving forward.

In terms of current trends in the reprofessionalisation of medicine, recent statements from the Ministry of Economic Development of the Russian Federation suggest that the state would like to transfer some of its regulatory functions to professional associations (Moskovskaya et al, 2013). Nonetheless, it has not provided the means to do this and appears only to see self-regulation in terms of partial autonomy from the state without widespread professional control or discretion. This is likely to limit the potential impact of the National Medical Chamber, a new professionalising organisation formed in 2010 from several medical bodies, including the Russian Association of Private Medical Practitioners (Mansurov and Yurchenko, 2011). This organisation is at present endeavouring to obtain legally enshrined professional market closure, including compulsory membership of a self-regulatory register and greater medical control of qualifications. While it has had a positive relationship with the government since its foundation, the state seems to have encouraged the Doctors' Society of Russia, a less challenging body, to draw away membership from the National Medical Chamber (Moskovskaya et al, 2013). The future, therefore, hinges on the degree to which the state will cede power to medicine, alongside other developing professions, in the evolving market system (Iarskaia-Smirnova and Abramov, 2016). This currently seems improbable given the weakness of professionalising associations in medicine and the Tsarist and Soviet legacy of state centrism that is writ large under Putin (Zimmerman, 2014). Either way, though, it remains important that the new Russia puts in place regulatory mechanisms in medicine that will more effectively protect the health of the public.

Acknowledgement
Sincere thanks are given to Roman Abramov, Deputy Head of Department and Associate Professor at the National Research University Higher School of Economics in Moscow, Russia, for his comments on an earlier version of this chapter.

References
Allsop, J., Mansurov, V. and Saks, M. (1999) 'Working conditions and earning options of physicians in the Russian Federation: a comparative case study', in Mansurov, V. (ed) *Russia Today: Sociological Outlook*, Moscow: Russian Society of Sociologists.

Bernstein, F., Burton, C. and Healey, D. (2010) 'Experts, expertise, and new histories of Soviet medicine', in Bernstein, F., Burton, C. and Healey, D. (eds) *Soviet Medicine: Culture, Practice and Science*, DeKalb, IL: Northern Illinois University Press.

Brown, J. (1987) 'The deprofessionalization of Soviet physicians: a reconsideration', *International Journal of Health Services* 17(1): 65-76.

Coulter, I., Katrova, L. and Maida, C. (2006) 'What impact does the transition from communist to post-communist society have on professions: from de-professionalization to re-professionalization?', paper presented at the International Sociological Association World Congress on The Quality of Social Existence in a Globalising World, Durban, South Africa, July.

Davidova, N., Manning, N., Palosua, H. and Koivusalo, M. (2009) 'Social policy and the health crisis in the new Russia', in Manning, N. and Tikhonova, N. (eds) *Health and Health Care in the New Russia*, Farnham: Ashgate.

Davis, C. (1989) 'The Soviet health system: A national health service in a socialist society', in Field, M. (ed) *Success and Crisis in National Health Systems: A Comparative Approach*, London: Sage.

Field, M. (1957) *Doctor and Patient in Soviet Russia*, Cambridge, MA: Harvard University Press.

Field, M. (1967) *Soviet Socialized Medicine: An Introduction*, New York, NY: Free Press.

Field, M. (2000) 'Soviet medicine', in Cooter, R. and Pickstone, J. (eds) *Medicine in the Twentieth Century*, Amsterdam: Harwood Academic Publishers.

Field, M. and Twigg, J. (eds) (2000) *Russia's Torn Safety Nets: Health and Social Welfare During the Transition*, Basingstoke: Palgrave Macmillan.

Frieden, N. (1981) *Russian Physicians in an Era of Reform and Revolution, 1856-1905*, Princeton, NJ: Princeton University Press.

Fry, D. J. (2012) *Medicine in Three Societies: A Comparison of Medical Care in the USSR, USA and the UK*, London: Springer.

Geltzer, A. (2009) 'When the standards aren't standards: evidence-based medicine in the Russian context', *Social Science and Medicine* 68(3): 526-32.

Geyer, M. and Fitzpatrick, S. (eds) (2009) *Beyond Totalitarianism: Stalinism and Nazism Compared*, New York, NY: Cambridge University Press.

Harden, J. (2001) '"Mother Russia" at work: gender divisions in the medical profession', *European Journal of Women's Studies* 8(2): 181-99.

Henderson, J. (2011) *The Constitution of the Russian Federation: A Contextual Analysis*, Oxford: Hart Publishing.

Hosking, G. (2012) *Russia and the Russians: From Earliest Times to the Present* (2nd edition), London: Penguin Books.

Hyde, G. (1974) *The Soviet Health Service: A Historical and Comparative Study*, London: Lawrence & Wishart.

Iarskaia-Smirnova, E. and Abramov, R. (2016) 'Professions and professionalization in Russia', in Dent, M., Bourgeault, I. L., Denis, J.-L. and Kuhlmann, E. (eds) *The Routledge Companion to the Professions and Professionalism*, London: Routledge.

Iarskaia-Smirnova, E. and Romanov, P. (2008) 'Culture matters: integration of folk medicine into healthcare in Russia', in Kuhlmann, E. and Saks, M. (eds) *Rethinking Professional Governance: International Directions in Healthcare*, Bristol: Policy Press.

Kuhlmann, E. and Saks, M. (2008) 'Changing patterns of health professional governance', in Kuhlmann, E. and Saks, M. (eds) *Rethinking Professional Governance: International Directions in Healthcare*, Bristol: Policy Press.

McClelland, C. (1991) *The German Experience of Professionalization: Modern Learned Professions and their Organizations from the Early Nineteenth Century to the Hitler Era*, Cambridge: Cambridge University Press.

McKinlay, J. and Arches, J. (1985) 'Towards the proletarianization of physicians', *International Journal of Health Services* 18: 161-95.

Mansurov, V., Luksha, O., Allsop, J. and Saks, M. (2004) 'The Anglo-American and Russian sociology of the professions: comparisons and perspectives', *Knowledge, Work and Society* 2(2): 27-48.

Mansurov, V. and Yurchenko, O. (2011) 'Professional ideology of altruism of Russian medical practitioners', *International Journal of Organizations* 6: 7-27.

Moskovskaya, A., Oberemko, O., Silaeva, V., Popova, I., Nazarova, I., Peshkova, O. and Chemysheva, M. (2013) *Development of Professional Associations in Russia: Research into Institutional Framework, Self-regulation Activity, and Barriers to Professionalization*, working paper BRP 26/SOC/2013, Moscow: Higher School of Economics.

Navarro, V. (1977) *Social Security and Medicine in the USSR: A Marxist Critique*, Lexington, MA: Lexington Books.

Nazarova, I. (2009) 'Access to health care and self-care', in Manning, N. and Tikhonova, N. (eds) *Health and Health Care in the New Russia*, Farnham: Ashgate.

OECD (Organisation for Economic Co-operation and Development) (2012) *Reviews of Health Systems: Russian Federation*, Paris: OECD Publishing.

Porter, R. (2002) *Blood and Guts: A Short History of Medicine*, London: Allen Lane.

Prisyazhnyuk, D. and Sadykov, R. (2012) 'The transformation of the medical profession in the context of Russian healthcare reforms', paper presented at the European Sociological Association Conference on Professions and Social Inequalities, University of Helsinki, Finland, May.

Read, C. (1990) *Culture and Power in Revolutionary Russia: The Intelligentsia and the Transition from Tsarism to Communism*, Basingstoke: Macmillan.

Ryan, M. (1989) *Doctors and the State in the Soviet Union*, Basingstoke: Macmillan.

Saks, M. (1995) *Professions and the Public Interest: Medical Power, Altruism and Alternative Medicine*, London: Routledge.

Saks, M. (2015) *The Professions, State and the Market: Medicine in Britain, the United States and Russia*, London: Routledge.

Saks, M. (2016) 'Review of theories of professions, organizations and society: neo-Weberianism, neo-institutionalism and eclecticism', *Journal of Professions and Organization* 3(2): 170-87.

Sakwa, R. (2010) *Communism in Russia: An Interpretative Essay*, Basingstoke: Palgrave Macmillan.

Sakwa, R. (2014) *Putin Redux: Power and Contradiction in Contemporary Russia*, London: Routledge.

Salo, E. (2009) 'Studying the activity of professional associations of traditional medicine in Moscow', in Mansurov, V. (ed) *European Society or European Societies: A View from Russia*, Moscow: Russian Society of Sociologists.

Savelli, M. and Marks, S. (eds) (2015) *Psychiatry in Communist Europe*, Basingstoke: Palgrave Macmillan.

Schecter, K. (1997) 'Physicians and health care in the former Soviet Union', in Shuval, J. and Bernstein, J. (eds) *Immigrant Physicians: Former Soviet Doctors in Israel, Canada and the United States*, Westport, CT: Praeger Publishers.

Service, R. (2009) *The Penguin History of Modern Russia: From Tsarism to the Twenty-First Century* (3rd edition), London: Penguin Books.

Sirotkina, I. (2010) 'Toward a Soviet psychiatry: war and the organization of mental health care in revolutionary Russia', in Bernstein, F., Burton, C. and Healey, D. (eds) *Soviet Medicine: Culture, Practice and Science*, DeKalb, IL: Northern Illinois University Press.

Solomon, S. and Hutchinson, J. (eds) (1990) *Health and Society in Revolutionary Russia*, Bloomington, IN: Indiana University Press.

Tulchinsky, T. H. and Varavikova, E. A. (2014) *The New Public Health* (3rd edition), Salt Lake City, UT: Academic Press.

Twigg, J. (2001) 'Russian health care reform at the regional level: status and impact', *Post-Soviet Geography and Economics* 42(3): 202-19.

Twigg, J. (2002) 'Health care reform in Russia: a survey of head doctors and insurance administrators', *Social Science and Medicine* 55(12): 2253-4.

Yurchenko, O. (2004) 'A sociological analysis of professionalisation of orthodox and alternative medicine in Russia', unpublished PhD thesis, De Montfort University.

Yurchenko, O. and Saks, M. (2006) 'The social integration of complementary and alternative medicine in official health care in Russia', *Knowledge, Work and Society* 4: 107-27.

Zimmerman, W. (2014) *Ruling Russia: Authoritarianism from the Revolution to Putin*, Princeton, NJ: Princeton University Press.

EIGHT

Patterns of medical oversight and regulation in Canada

Humayun Ahmed, Adalsteinn Brown and Mike Saks

Introduction

As medical professionals, physicians in Canada have among the greatest extent of self-regulatory powers internationally. They have gained what can be described in neo-Weberian terms as a dominant form of exclusionary social closure in a competitive marketplace. Here their interests have prevailed in so far as they have managed across Canadian provinces and territories to create a legally enshrined group of insiders based on registration, with distinctive market advantages over outsiders (Saks, 2010). As this chapter will argue, the consequence of this social closure has been to make this a group, which – while differentiated by specialism and other factors and subject to variations in its statutory underpinning across provinces and territories – has generally managed to increase its income, status and power in the occupational pecking order. This has been a common pattern in the modern Western world, although in Canada this standing has been arguably more open to challenge by public opinion. This is likely to have occurred in Canada, as compared with the United States (US), because of scandals around professional discipline (Donovan, 2016) and the policy constraints surrounding an affordable and universal health care system (Nadeau et al, 2014).

Whether or not this professional self-regulation in medicine and the gains to its beneficiaries are justified and effective in terms of the public interest has increasingly been the subject of a debate driven by both internal and external actors, including physicians themselves, the state, citizens, the popular media and multinational corporations (Kuhlmann and Saks, 2008). There is no doubt, though, about the political drive for a healthier Canadian society, including through medical practice (Hutchison et al, 2011; Deber and Mah, 2014). As a result of this, medicine has become more focused on quality and the reformulation of quality as process and outcomes rather than just inputs or structures, and in the case of Ontario as an inclusive notion of health system performance. Moreover, critics as well as the public advocate increased regulatory engagement in physician oversight, lay community contribution to and awareness of governance, and analysis of the inadequacies of the current health care system. To some extent, therefore, medical regulation has been increasingly incisively analysed – not just in the wake of the 1960s and 1970s counterculture, but also beyond (Saks, 2000). The questions of why medicine in particular is self-regulated and how regulation is likely to evolve in future in a highly differentiated division of health care labour have therefore often been the subjects of academic exploration in Canada and elsewhere (see, for example, Allsop and Saks, 2003; Cruess and Cruess, 2005).

However, relatively little work has thus far been undertaken to evaluate the performance of presently implemented regulatory structures in medicine (as highlighted by, for example, Chamberlain, 2015). Although such structures have been studied in Canada both nationally (see, for example, Wenghofer, 2015) and in international context (as illustrated by Allsop and Jones, 2008), and there is some research more generally on factors affecting physician performance (see, for instance, Wenghofer et al, 2009), much the same can be said of Canada itself. Logically, though, if changes to regulation are to be proposed, it is necessary to understand how well the current regulatory framework is performing. In order to evaluate current performance, we must first understand the goals and standards of behaviour and core medical skills that regulatory bodies expect of themselves and doctors in Canada. These standards are largely described or implicit in the charters, legislation and other foundational or core documentation of medical colleges and boards that are responsible for licensing and overseeing doctors' competence and fitness to practise. Nonetheless, although this documentation is publicly available, it has not as yet been coherently analysed in Canada.

Using original research and recognising that informal mechanisms of physician control such as the colleague boycott also exist (Rosenthal, 1995), this chapter will seek to overview the pattern of standards and regulatory goals and the various formal mechanisms that are in place for doctors in Canada. In so doing, it will sketch out how provincial and territorial medical colleges, including their governance mechanisms, explicitly and implicitly understand, describe and implement their own standards of performance, and provide a commentary on the extent to which the engagement of colleges with quality assurance fits with the definition of quality that has emerged within the medical field in recent years and the more general public interest.

Although Canada has physician oversight at both federal and provincial/territorial levels, the focus is on colleges in the provinces and territories for the purpose of this analysis, for three reasons. The first of these is that, although the federal bodies – the Canadian College of Family Physicians and the Royal College of Physicians and Surgeons of Canada – certify physicians' competence on completion of their training programmes and over their career, the provincial and territorial bodies have a broader scope of oversight and their certification is required for physician billing and other aspects of practice in each jurisdiction. This dual certification system exists because the Canadian and Royal Colleges differ from the provincial/territorial colleges and boards in terms of the types of assessments they provide. Specifically, the federal bodies:

- define the requirements for specialty education across medical, surgical and laboratory medicine;
- are the primary point of certification for both locally and internationally trained physicians, conducting the federal certifying examinations that physicians must pass prior to obtaining a provincial or territorial licence;
- administer continuing professional development via the Maintenance of Certification Program, a mandatory programme that awards credits to physicians who demonstrate continued investment in professional advancement.

The Royal College also formally states on its website that it 'sets standards for professional and ethical conduct among its members' (Royal College of Physicians and Surgeons of Canada, 2016), but this is largely in the form of advocating adherence to the Canadian Medical Association (CMA) Code of Ethics and accompanying documentation rather than drafting novel standards of behaviour. By contrast, the provincial and territorial colleges largely play licensing and disciplinary roles, with the exception of the Collège des Médecins du Québec, which shares responsibility for certifying physicians with the Royal College.

The second reason for the focus on colleges in the provinces and territories is that health care in Canada remains largely a function of the provincial/territorial governments, including physician oversight bodies, so major changes in how health care systems are responding to physician oversight are most likely to be seen at this level. Finally, provincial and territorial medical colleges in Canada have not been as thoroughly analysed as their analogous structures in the US, which may help to enable future cross-national comparisons based on this analysis (see, for instance, Starr, 1984; Saks, 2015b). This brings us to the methodology used in the analysis.

The methodology employed in the study

Since relatively little work has been undertaken on Canadian medical regulatory bodies' expectations of their own standards, two sets of methods for the review in this chapter were brought together. First, scoping methods were used to identify the full range of relevant materials published by Canadian regulatory bodies, such as legislation, charters and publicly available articles. The scoping review component of this work predominantly followed the protocol specified in Arksey and O'Malley (2005), updated by Levac and colleagues (2010). Content analysis was then employed to critically evaluate the texts for evidence of regulatory bodies' expectations of their own regulatory standards. Combining these methods, answers were sought to the following questions: What methods currently exist for medical professional oversight and regulation in Canada and how do medical regulatory bodies understand their own performance?

To develop the scoping question, several texts relevant to this regulatory space were consulted. Specifically, given the neo-Weberian context of this chapter, several works discussing health professional regulation from this perspective were consulted, such as Allsop and Saks (2003). Recent reviews of Canadian regulatory practice in medicine were also examined to gain a sense of the structure of the Canadian regulatory landscape (for example, Shaw et al, 2009; Horsley et al, 2016). Next, a search strategy and selected keywords were defined regarding Canadian medical regulation at the provincial/territorial and federal levels. These primarily returned the websites of provincial and territorial medical colleges and federal oversight structures, prompting further examination of individual bodies. Regulatory bodies concerned with the management of health professions strictly outside the scope of medicine and surgery (for example, dentistry, psychiatry and nursing) were excluded in the interests of defining the single regulatory landscape on which this chapter is centred – although interprofessional comparisons are of course important, not least given the interconnectedness of the health care division of labour.

In this regard, it should also be stressed that the focus of this chapter is on the regulation of allopathic rather than complementary and alternative medicine as this has its own interlinked conflict-based dynamics from a neo-Weberian perspective (see, among others,

Saks, 2015a). Within this framework, the websites of all 14 Canadian provincial/territorial colleges were examined in order to isolate statements of outcomes and standards. Outcomes are defined here as goals upon which regulatory medical colleges wish to tangibly deliver, often in the form of specific materials or services (for instance, providing information to patients and equipping physicians with continuing education programmes). Standards are defined here as principles by which the colleges aim to operate in fulfilling these outcomes (for example, transparency, professional development and commitment to self-regulation). The content of websites rather than printed sources was analysed because college publications are now virtually all online. This is illustrated by the case of the College of Physicians and Surgeons of Ontario, whose annual report, patient resources, newsletters, task force reports and new member welcome information are all digitised, with no allusions made to printed copies.

Each regulatory body's website was reviewed and relevant details of their content were recorded. Targeted site searches were also performed for certain details, including determining whether or not transparency was suggested as a commitment of a given body. These details were comparatively reviewed and emerging themes were identified, which were framed as commitments. Tables were created featuring both the isolated themes and the regulatory bodies analysed. Each regulatory body was then examined in terms of its stated dedication to each commitment. If regulatory body documentation revealed clear textual evidence of a commitment to a given outcome or standard, then a 'Yes' was assigned. If regulatory body documentation did not mention a standard or outcome, a 'No' was assigned. Concurrently, provincial and territorial legislation was searched to elicit how self-defined regulatory body commitments aligned with the legal obligations imposed on those bodies by Acts such as the Regulated Health Professions Act (Ontario) 1991.

It is important to note that the themes isolated in the analysis were derived from colleges' self-presentation within their own documentation rather than from the core legislation to which they are accountable. In addition to their own standards, colleges espouse several laws, many of which differ between jurisdictions, but most of which share fundamental tenets as to how colleges should actually operate. One core legal mandate of all colleges is registration. While this, for instance, is mandated under the Health Professions Act in Alberta 2000 and British Columbia 1996 as compared with the Medicine Act in Ontario 1991, all Canadian provincial/territorial college legislation stresses the need for colleges to act as registrars, and all Canadian colleges currently register physicians. Provincial and territorial variation aside, the legislation also usually specifies rules for college council composition and performance via a set of by-laws, and stresses the need for quality assurance, interprofessional collaboration and strong professional ethics as core components of college behaviour.

As much as the core aspects of the legislation are consistent across the provinces and the territories, certain aspects of the law remain unique to particular jurisdictions. As an example, the Health Professions Act of British Columbia 1996 significantly elaborates on the role of health profession corporations, and why they may be problematic, but this is not a commonly addressed theme within the legislative guidelines of other provinces and territories. Certain other provinces and territories did not detail the legislation lying behind their commitments at all: the Nunavut Department of Health and Social Services, for instance, avoids referring to legislation on its website. Some territory organisations, such as the Department of Health and Social Services, also featured more legislation than was found on websites in the provinces – including in relation to Acts specifically detailing emergency medicine, Aboriginal recognition and health information.

In sum, therefore, while outcomes and standards could be explored in more detail in relation to the legislation described above – which is largely consistent across the provinces and territories at its core – the focus of the methodology employed in this chapter is on the variability inherent in what colleges say they will do rather than what they are actually legally mandated to do.

The results of the study

A summation of some of the most prevalent themes that can be isolated from medical college rather than legislative websites is set out in Table 8.1. Overall, the outcomes mandated by law and the standards emphasised by the colleges do align, but intercollege stated or implied adherence to commitments varies. In Table 8.1, the orientation of all 14 provincial and territorial medical colleges (including the Federation of Health Regulatory Colleges of Ontario) is described with respect to outcomes and standards – where, as previously mentioned, 'Yes' indicates that the college overtly commits to the standard, while 'No' indicates otherwise. These outcomes and standards are not necessarily derived directly from the legislation, but relate to generalised positions present in college web materials. The outcomes and standards featured were selected on the basis of being either explicitly stated within or readily derivable from colleges' online documentation. An example of this would be 'enforcing practice standards', behaviour that was frequently committed to explicitly. On the other hand, 'general health information provision' was not often mentioned, but was nonetheless a recurrent focus of college websites, and can thus be inferred to be an outcome to which colleges implicitly aspire.

As Table 8.1 indicates, Canadian provincial and territorial colleges appear to understand their performance as a variable combination of adherence to standards and fulfilment of outcomes. Their commitments can broadly be subdivided into two major categories in terms of the themes of this book: patient-centred commitments and physician-centred commitments.

Patient-centred commitments

The first main category of outcomes and standards to which regulatory bodies commit is typically patient-centred. As the Federation of Health Regulatory Colleges of Ontario (FHRCO) notes, 'the first responsibility of each college is to [the patient]', and 'colleges have the responsibility and legal authority to protect [the patient]'. Similarly, the website of the College of Physicians and Surgeons of British Columbia states that 'the College's overriding interest is the protection and safety of patients', and more broadly that 'regulation ... is based on the foundation that the College must act first and foremost in the interest of the public'. Interestingly, attention to consumerism permeates some colleges' commitments to patient-centredness: the Colleges of Physicians and Surgeons of New Brunswick and Manitoba, for example, both state that their mandates are to 'protect the public as consumers of medical care', alluding to the fact that patients' self-interests may not necessarily align with the interests of physicians and the market.

It should be noted that what strictly constitutes quality in terms of patient-centredness is poorly defined. Many provincial and territorial colleges, as already mentioned, state that their mandate is to 'protect' the public, foster the 'safety' of patients and increase the 'competence' of medical professionals, but what increased protection, safety and competence look like is not clearly delineated. By contrast, the Institute of Medicine (2001), for instance, has a relatively clear definition of quality, with six key dimensions that include patient-centredness and safety. And even if we were to accept the relatively unelaborated terminology of 'protection', 'safety' and 'competence' that the provincial and territorial colleges use, these terms are not synonymous with a comprehensive, current understanding of quality.

Table 8.1: Canadian medical regulatory bodies: summation of self-presented outcomes and standards of provincial and territorial colleges

Regulatory body	General health information provision	Disciplinary information provision	Patient transparency	Connecting patients to physicians	Setting practice standards	Enforcing practice standards	Physician registration	Practice standard publication	Continuing physician education	Acknowledging the importance of self-regulation	Core value declaration	Lawfulness
College of Physicians and Surgeons of Alberta	No	No	No	Yes	Yes	Yes	Yes	Yes	Yes	Yes	Yes	No
College of Physicians and Surgeons of British Columbia	Yes	No	Yes	Yes	Yes	Yes	Yes	Yes	Yes	Yes	Yes	Yes
College of Physicians and Surgeons of Manitoba	Yes	No	No	Yes	No	Yes	Yes	Yes	No	Yes	No	Yes
College of Physicians and Surgeons of New Brunswick	No	No	No	Yes	Yes	Yes	Yes	Yes	No	No	No	No

Regulatory body	General health information provision	Disciplinary information provision	Patient transparency	Connecting patients to physicians	Setting practice standards	Enforcing practice standards	Physician registration	Practice standard publication	Continuing physician education	Acknowledging the importance of self-regulation	Core value declaration	Lawfulness
College of Physicians and Surgeons of Newfoundland and Labrador	Yes	No	No	Yes	Yes	Yes	Yes	Yes	No	Yes	No	Yes
Department of Health and Social Services (Nunavut)	Yes	No	No	No	No	Yes	Yes	No	No	No	No	No
College of Physicians and Surgeons of Nova Scotia	No	Yes	Yes	Yes	Yes	Yes	Yes	Yes	Yes	Yes	Yes	Yes
Department of Health and Social Services (Northwest Territories)	Yes	No	No	No	No	No	Yes	No	No	No	No	Yes
College of Physicians and Surgeons of Ontario	No	Yes	Yes	Yes	Yes	Yes	Yes	Yes	Yes	Yes	Yes	Yes

Regulatory body	General health information provision	Disciplinary information provision	Patient transparency	Connecting patients to physicians	Setting practice standards	Enforcing practice standards	Physician registration	Practice standard publication	Continuing physician education	Acknowledging the importance of self-regulation	Core value declaration	Lawfulness
Federation of Health Regulatory Colleges of Ontario (FHRCO)	Yes	No	Yes	No	Yes	No	No	Yes	No	Yes	Yes	Yes
College of Physicians and Surgeons of Prince Edward Island	No	No	No	Yes	Yes	Yes	Yes	Yes	No	No	Yes	Yes
Collège des Médecins du Québec	No	No	No	Yes	Yes	Yes	Yes	Yes	Yes	Yes	No	Yes
College of Physicians and Surgeons of Saskatchewan	Yes	Yes	Yes	Yes	Yes	Yes	Yes	Yes	No	Yes	Yes	Yes
Yukon Medical Council	Yes	No	No	Yes	Yes	Yes	Yes	Yes	No	No	Yes	Yes

Thus, simply ensuring that patients are not harmed and that the competence of medical professionals is satisfactory does not constitute ensuring that truly high-quality care is provided. Patient engagement and education, holistic healing from a biopsychosocial perspective, interdisciplinary initiatives and the integration of novel technologies are further examples of quality considerations not encompassed by the three criteria mentioned here.

As part of their patient-centred commitments, many regulatory bodies aim to provide patients with generalised information about their health care. Approximately 57% (8/14) of all college websites, for example, feature informational articles regarding a range of health care-related topics – such as health care consumer rights, informed consent, medical record access, personal health information use and the medical profession. The College of Physicians and Surgeons of Newfoundland and Labrador, for instance, has a 'For the Public' section featuring a patient information article concerning opioid drugs. Similar 'For the Public' sections exist in Alberta, British Columbia and Ontario. As a more comprehensive example, Nunavut's Department of Health and Social Services, which is essentially the territory's regulatory college, has two subsections of its website devoted to public information: the first, entitled 'Programs', has information about how to maintain health (for instance, mental health, oral health and immunisation) and prevent and treat a range of diseases (including communicable and chronic diseases), while the second, entitled 'Healthy Living', briefs readers on exercise, eating, sexual health, tobacco reduction and emotional wellbeing. There are also less comprehensive examples:

- the College of Physicians and Surgeons of Manitoba, for instance, features a single Lyme disease information sheet and no other articles;
- the College of Physicians and Surgeons of Saskatchewan does not feature many patient-facing links, but does feature health card procural information;
- the Yukon Medical Council similarly features health care accessibility information but no general health care articles.

While these articles form a significant component of some colleges' websites, 43% (6/14) of provincial and territorial colleges do not feature them at all, indicating the variability in the extent to which colleges engage in public health care information dissemination. However, interestingly there was no information on physician performance in the patient-centred quality dimension available on any of the sites.

Patients can also utilise regulatory bodies to seek out more physician-specific information. They can confirm that a physician is registered with a college (that is, legally entitled to practise and use a professional title) and learn about elements of the professional record – for instance, suspensions of licences and results of disciplinary proceedings – of their health care provider. However, only 21% (3/14) of provincial and territorial medical colleges allow patients to access disciplinary information directly. In other words, while there has been a trend towards providing more physician qualification information to patients in certain other areas of the world such as the United Kingdom, such a trend is not as yet evident in Canada at the provincial and territorial level as only a minority of colleges commit to releasing physicians' past performance records. These are the Colleges of Physicians and Surgeons of Nova Scotia, Ontario and Saskatchewan, which all permit members of the public to retrieve a physician's registration status and disciplinary record via a name-based search. Providing patients with physician-specific disciplinary information may help in furthering regulatory bodies' commitments in relation not only to information dissemination, but also to physician accountability maintenance: if patients can readily access data about physicians' histories of compliance with standards of care, then practitioners may become more likely to perform to standards in their self-interest. This may be especially important in light of the fact that failure to discipline doctors in a way that seems proportionate to their offences has led to substantial public challenges. In Ontario, for example, the registrar of the College of Physicians and Surgeons of Ontario has publicly condemned its own independent disciplinary panel for inappropriately light punishment in sexual abuse cases (Gallant, 2016).

However, within the context of all this information sharing, regulatory bodies seem to rely on patient initiative. They do this by presenting themselves as assuming a responsive rather than an anticipatory role in physician oversight in a number of ways. First, the fact that regulatory bodies primarily disseminate information via websites and other passive vehicles presupposes that patients will know enough about the medical profession to understand where to take their complaints, concerns and questions, given that these tools are retrievable only by those who know enough to search for them using the right terms. Second, most of the language utilised on regulatory body websites reinforces the notion that the patient will be the initiator of patient–college contact. For example, websites suggest that 'by contacting a college', patients can obtain information, ask questions and report concerns and complaints. In another example, the FHRCO tells patients that:

> You can learn if someone is actually a registered professional by checking with the appropriate college. Each college has an online listing ... which you can search.... If you can't locate that individual on the registry, alerting the college would prompt a closer look. You can also call the college to ask about any of their registered professionals.

This latter wording makes it clear that, if the patient does not establish contact, regulatory help may not arrive. Most colleges do not appear to have well-defined methods of initiating contact with patients: their websites make no mention of outreach efforts geared explicitly at soliciting patient experiences, or even awareness efforts geared at disseminating knowledge of the existence of regulatory bodies. The wealth of patient- or public-focused information present on college websites would appear to suggest that regulatory body documentation targets individual health care consumers, and while meaningful dialogue with both patients and the public has recently been advocated, the initiation of patient–board dialogue is not directly addressed as a commitment. Instead, it seems to have been left as the responsibility of the patient, who, paradoxically, may not be sufficiently aware of the existence of regulatory bodies to access and use this carefully curated information.

The FHRCO does engage in raising public awareness: 'We Care about Your Care', for example, is a campaign discussed in President Marshall Moleschi's 2014 letter to Eric Hoskins, Minister of Health and Long-Term Care, and aims to 'provide information to Ontarians about the health regulatory system' (FHRCO, 2015). The same letter also notes that the federation publishes publicly oriented information articles on a regular basis, citing a not-so-recent relatively information-sparse piece from April 2013. It also says that 'significant funds are dedicated to educating the public about their right to access information and that health regulation in Ontario is in the public interest', although no mention is made of how precisely these funds are utilised or how the term 'the public interest' is defined. Despite these statements, however, most patients remain unaware of the nature of health care regulation.

Regulatory bodies also seem to have a commitment to being transparent to patients where their own regulatory processes are concerned. About 43% (6/14) of provincial colleges mention 'transparency' somewhere on their websites, usually in the context of a need for transparency or clearly transparent measures of physician competence. The FHRCO, for example, notes that patients can contact a college to 'obtain information about [its] standards', and find out more about disciplinary decisions. More explicitly, the FHRCO also states that it and its member colleges 'share a commitment ... to transparency in the regulated health care system', and discusses measures it has taken – including through federation meetings and the Advisory Group for Regulatory Excellence policy research – to enhance transparency in recent years. Similarly, the College of Physicians and Surgeons of British Columbia mentions on its 'Mission, Mandate and Values' page that there is a need for 'registration, inquiry and discipline processes that are transparent'. The College of Physicians and Surgeons of Nova Scotia had a similar page, which has since been reconfigured to be more trust-related.

On the other hand, the College of Physicians and Surgeons of British Columbia advances transparency by holding 'open portions of ... board meetings' that the public can sit in on. Some regulatory bodies also practise transparency in a different sense – namely, by revealing concrete strategic goals to the public. The College of Physicians and Surgeons of British Columbia, for example, publicised its three-year strategic plan on its website. Similarly, the College of Physicians and Surgeons of Ontario publishes annual reports concerning its progress. The College of Physicians and Surgeons of Nova Scotia, in addition to defining transparency in its strategic themes, prioritises this value by asserting that it ensures that 'all College communications ... are written in plain language', important matters are communicated to the public and 'information is shared consistently'.

In another sense, as they often serve as creators of databases of registered practitioners, regulatory bodies can also act as connectors, bridging the gap between patients and physicians. Seventy-nine per cent (11/14) of colleges explicitly connect patients to physicians through physician search repositories. The FHRCO, for instance, notes that its website may be used to 'find a health care professional'. The College of Physicians and Surgeons of Ontario features a page called 'Doctors Search', which allows patients to instantly search for physicians, but is included chiefly for the purpose of locating physicians to seek care, not to understand the performance of these professionals. Other college websites, including the websites of the Colleges of Alberta, British Columbia, Manitoba, New Brunswick, Newfoundland and Labrador, Nova Scotia, Prince Edward Island, Quebec, Saskatchewan and, to some degree, the Yukon, feature similarly titled pages that serve parallel functions. It is unclear, though, how this functionality is related to the standards or goals for physicians defined in the colleges' materials.

Finally, and perhaps most importantly, regulatory bodies see the oversight of physicians as the primary part of their patient protection mandate. They fulfil this mandate by defining physician accountability. In particular, 79% (11/14) of colleges explicitly mention 'setting … standards and guidelines of practice and conduct' as their responsibility. However, regulatory bodies do not solely establish standards: 86% (12/14) of colleges also write that they should enforce them. As far as this is concerned, they seem to take more a reactive than a preventive stance: in other words, colleges do not demonstrate any defined methods of regularly evaluating the state of physician compliance, with enforcement usually only occurring in a disciplinary capacity. Essentially, 'enforcement' in the language of the regulatory college seems to be equivalent to a 'disciplinary response to non-compliance'.

To be sure, some regulatory bodies do mention attempts to enforce implementation of standards prior to any violation occurring by running quality assurance programmes. The College of Physicians and Surgeons of Ontario, for example, has set a goal of 'assessing every doctor every 10 years', and took steps towards this in 2015 by assessing 2,349 of the 34,124 physicians currently practising. For the most part, however, regulatory bodies do not concretely delineate goals in this respect, and enforcement seems to be limited to responding to patient concerns and complaints, collecting peer assessments from health care practitioners, and mediating patient–physician relationships when external intervention becomes necessary. As an example, the College of Physicians and Surgeons of Ontario includes both the Inquiries, Complaints and Reports Committee and the Discipline Committee, which act complementarily in investigating cases and enforcing disciplinary measures.

Physician-centred commitments

In terms of the second major category of physician-centred commitments, regulatory bodies are accountable for physician registration. In fact, in all but one of the provincial institutions featured – the FHRCO understandably was an exception, given that it is more of an oversight structure – physician registration was cited as a core responsibility. Since all physicians must be members of a regulatory college in order to practise medicine in their jurisdiction, regulatory bodies double as physician registrars. Besides carrying out physician registration, they provide information about the registration process, issue registration certificates and handle registration-related inquiries. Some 57% (8/14) of regulatory bodies also mention that they seek to demonstrate transparency to physicians. For example, some medical colleges showcase their by-laws – as well as the federal and provincial legislation relevant to their conduct – on their websites. The College of Physicians and Surgeons of Ontario, for instance, has a page called 'Legislation and By-Laws', which outlines the Regulated Health Professions Act 1991, the Medicine Act 1991 and the by-laws that govern its existence. Similar pages also exist on the websites of the Colleges of Manitoba, Nova Scotia, Prince Edward Island, Quebec, Saskatchewan and the Yukon.

Although not all regulatory bodies feature physician practice guidelines, 86% (12/14) of regulatory body websites do so – namely, a code of conduct, a code of ethics and/or clinical guidelines. A code of conduct – often the College of Physicians and Surgeons Association (CPSA) Code of Conduct, derived from the CMA Code of Ethics and complementary to the CPSA Standards of Practice – typically delineates behavioural and value standards for physicians such as accountability, confidentiality, respect for others and responsibility. It may, for example, include behaviours such as:

- accurate reporting;
- minimising discussion of patients' problems;
- complying with legislation;
- refraining from offensive, sexual and overly personal contact with co-workers and patients;
- avoiding discrimination;
- maintaining professional language;
- addressing breaches of conduct by other physicians;
- avoiding substance abuse that could interfere with patient care;
- prioritising patient safety.

By contrast, a code of ethics – usually in this case the CMA Code of Ethics – lays out both more precise standards of behaviour in certain situations, as well as broader, more value-based standards. It also relates to a wider range of areas, including research and decision making, and is more frequently updated (every five to six years necessarily). For example, the CMA Code of Ethics spans both such specific topics as how to initiate and dissolve a patient–physician relationship and such broad value standards as recognising one's own limitations as a physician. It elaborates too on decision making, research, and responsibilities to oneself, society and the profession, none of which are explicitly covered in certain other codes of conduct. Finally, clinical practice guidelines – for instance, the CPSA Standards of Practice – generally outline the minimum standards of professional behaviour and ethical conduct and include tangible, legally requisite behaviours across a range of specific situations. They encompass, among other things, what is required of the physician in cases of advertising, patient record retention, uninsured services, industrial applications, medical equipment, transfer of care, closing a practice and more tangible scenarios.

Each college makes use of a distinct combination of the aforementioned documents. The College of Physicians and Surgeons of Alberta – which, incidentally, boasts a particularly physician-friendly web presence, dedicating half of its online content to physicians alone – publishes all three documents. The Colleges of British Columbia, Manitoba, Newfoundland and Labrador, Ontario and Saskatchewan also either publish three distinct documents, or clearly allude to all three codes within one document. Some other colleges, such as the Colleges of New Brunswick and Prince Edward Island, delineate a code of ethics and practice guidelines, but define standards of misconduct rather than standards of conduct. Still other regions, such as Nova Scotia, Quebec and the Yukon, have no explicitly defined code of conduct. Finally, Nunavut and the Northwest Territories appear to rely solely on external legislation to set practice guidelines, referring only to the Medical on their web pages.

Regulatory bodies have also committed to physician continuing education. The FHRCO, for instance, notes that one of its responsibilities and legal authorities rests in 'developing programs to help members continually improve their skills and knowledge'. This is seen as a fundamental way to uphold the quality of care, and thus doubles as a patient protection-centred standard. The extent of these programmes, however, is not detailed on the publicly accessible parts of the FHRCO website: the only physician-targeted documents appearing on the site are the 'FHRCO Guide to Medical Directives and Delegation' and the 'FHRCO Interprofessional Collaboration (IPC) eTool'. Two physician-targeted workshops are also described: one is deemed 'basic' and the other 'advanced', although both centre on orienting physicians entering practice. This is the case with many other regulatory bodies; in fact only 36% (5/14) of colleges have some kind of tangible continuing education resources – or even make explicit reference to continuing education as a standard – on their websites.

Another physician-related commitment that many regulatory bodies have is less tangible than one might expect. This is the commitment to setting standards that can coexist with physician self-regulation.

Although policy makers in countries such as Britain have recently challenged the notion that medicine should be wholly self-regulated (Chamberlain, 2015), most regulatory bodies in Canada do not: the College of Physicians and Surgeons of Ontario, for example, acknowledges that 'doctors in Ontario have been granted a degree of authority for self-regulation under provincial law', and cites maintaining 'an effective system of self-governance' as one of its core mandates. Approximately 64% (9/14) of colleges explicitly acknowledge the need for self-regulation somewhere on their website.

Although they can be seen to protect patients and provide oversight of physicians, regulatory bodies also parallel and facilitate the evolution of the medical and regulatory professions, and around 21% (3/14) mention that some variant of advancing the medical profession is a commitment. In some instances, they initiate projects that serve to systemically enhance health care. The FHRCO, for instance, has directly involved itself in advancing electronic health through schemes such as the Connecting GTA project, a new electronic medical records system to be launched in community health centres, and a pilot project involving patient–physician computer tablet communication. Regulatory bodies also work in tandem with the government. The College of Physicians and Surgeons of Ontario, for example, explicitly notes that it is involved in the management of 'a number of government programs', including conducting a quality assurance assessment of Independent Health Facilities and Methadone Programs.

Having said this, most regulatory bodies set standards of behaviour not solely for physicians, but also for themselves. Regulatory bodies more often than not have a set of core ethical values that they display on their websites – approximately 57% (8/14), according to the analysis here. Commonly cited values include integrity, accountability, and cooperation/collaboration with other authorities, the government, academic institutions and the public. Other cited principles include leadership, justice, principledness, progressiveness and service orientation. Many regulatory bodies also hold themselves explicitly accountable in terms of operating within the confines of the law, with 79% (11/14) of colleges explicitly mentioning adherence to legality as important to their functioning. Thus, the College of Physicians and Surgeons of British Columbia notes that it 'regulates the practice of medicine under the authority of provincial law' and that it responds to not only incompetent and unethical practice, but also illegal practice. Similar statements are made on the websites of the Colleges of Manitoba, Newfoundland and Labrador, Nova Scotia, the Northwest

Territories, Ontario, Prince Edward Island, Quebec, Saskatchewan and the Yukon.

A final standard of behaviour that is nearly universally espoused by the colleges is adverse event reporting. The Colleges of Alberta, British Columbia, Manitoba, New Brunswick, Ontario, Prince Edward Island, Quebec and Saskatchewan all mention the need to report adverse events (for example, patient deaths and drug reactions) either in their core documentation or in press releases. However, the Colleges of Newfoundland and Labrador, Nova Scotia and the Yukon, and the Departments of Health of Nunavut and the Northwest Territories, do not overtly mention the need for adverse event reporting. This highlights the variability between provincial and territorial colleges in their physician-centred commitments, which can be viewed as complementing their patient-centred commitments.

Conclusion

Health care self-regulation in medicine is typically seen by neo-Weberian social scientists as a means of exclusionary social closure, through which physicians can ensure that they retain control of their working environment in accord with their interests (see, among others, Saks, 2015b). This chapter set about looking at what the variations between provinces and territories are in the goals and standards of behaviour that can be used to justify closure and particularly how the various medical regulatory colleges see their role in justifying closure. Overall, the nature of the physician-oriented commitments made by the provincial/territorial colleges is consistent with the argument that they are seeking to secure professional self-regulation in an ongoing fashion and to capture the market, and thus accords with much of the neo-Weberian literature in this field. College documentation overwhelmingly reflects the importance of setting and enforcing behavioural practice standards, connecting physicians to patients, and abiding by legal standards, all of which can help to ensure that physicians remain self-regulated and thus retain control of their market. Conversely, objectives around improving patient experience are common, but have little detail and largely rely on the patient's initiation of processes – even in cases where they do not unduly compromise physicians – as, for example, the provision of information about physician disciplinary records and general health care information dissemination – which is much less consistently noted in publicly available materials from the colleges.

This said, despite all provincial and territorial colleges being governed by the Medical Act and Regulations and the CMA Code of Ethics, by which they should therefore abide, colleges' own expectations of performance seem to differ significantly. Some colleges express behavioural standards that others lack entirely. The degree to which different commitments manifest themselves in different provincial/territorial jurisdictions may reflect diverse patterns of reliance on market forces in specific parts of Canada. For example, in Nunavut, significant emphasis is placed on disseminating information that helps people to care for themselves. Here the Department of Health and Social Services has a website that includes information about health and disease, geared to helping people to do this – which could in some respects be seen as standing counter to physicians' market prospects. This jurisdiction also houses very few doctors (some 144 family doctors in 2012, many of them on short-term contracts) (Dawson, 2013), suggesting perhaps that there is less pressure than in other provinces and territories to drive patients to seek medical care, allowing more focus on patient-executed preventive measures than on patient recruitment. However, given that these college roles are described in largely abstract fashion and the descriptions themselves may have an ideological function, it is difficult to gauge whether or not there is actual variability in the work carried out by these colleges.

Regardless of cause, this variability in implied goals suggests that the Canadian medical regulatory system has a notion of performance that is not easy to measure, and that is not presently measured. While, for example, many colleges suggest that they are responsible for continuing education programmes, no such programmes have as yet been implemented Canada-wide. Similarly, although colleges acknowledge that it is important to routinely inspect doctors for quality assurance purposes, most jurisdictions have not implemented periodic assessment programmes. For instance, the College of Physicians and Surgeons of Ontario has only now set the objective of assessing every doctor every 10 years. While many colleges appear to emphasise the importance of ensuring that practising physicians are disciplined in the event that they fail to fulfil minimal practice standards in the sense of either core skills or core behavioural competence, little attention seems to be dedicated to proactively advancing quality assurance, with colleges relying on patients to bring forward concerns retrospectively rather than prospectively enforcing inspection routines. This is exemplified by the fact that most of the discipline committee decisions discussed in the news releases of the College of Physicians and Surgeons of Ontario appeared to unfold in response to complaints, with no proactive attempt at validating these physicians' practices before the complaints were issued. That one doctor's offence unfolded in 1979 and his practice was not thoroughly explored until 2011/12 highlights the degree to which doctors are not routinely inspected.

The fact that many of these commitments are formalised but seem to lack a clear demonstration of active implementation suggests that regulatory colleges have been somewhat lenient when it comes to quality assurance, and this makes it more difficult to justify social closure from the viewpoint of the public. This is particularly important in a market context where the definition of quality and expectations of the health care system have expanded far beyond the expectations typical of colleges in terms of competent and ethical practice, where the need for integration with more complex teams of providers has become clearer. Moreover, the absence of engagement by the colleges in policy tools around quality such as performance reporting and performance management – which have become hallmarks of New Public Management approaches to policy (Dent et al, 2004) – have led to a situation where new organisations have moved into the arena where they challenge the role of colleges and ultimately their ability to maintain social closure.

Quality councils or agencies are one particularly common new entrant in Canada. They currently exist in Alberta, British Columbia, Manitoba, New Brunswick, Ontario, Quebec and Saskatchewan. The Canadian Patient Safety Institute also exists to coordinate a range of health sectors. While these organisations do not precisely duplicate the roles of regulatory colleges, they do begin to intersect with the work that regulatory colleges and physicians are doing, and can be seen as alternative accountability structures that create conflict for existing regulatory bodies. As such, they point from a neo-Weberian perspective increasingly towards a neo-institutional frame of reference, in which medicine as a profession is one among other institutions competing in an ecological system, including numerous other bodies such as the state and citizens (Saks, 2016). What is most important in the Canadian context is that this political interface results in clear and sustainable benefits for both the individual patient and the public interest – a wider and sometimes non-commensurate concept (Saks, 1995). Practically, this means that the influence of colleges is likely to decline, particularly if the new entrants are able to promise more effective professional oversight and more inclusive approaches to the health system that permit simpler delegation of expert oversight away from ministries of health. Indeed, recent calls for increased oversight and new focused forms of oversight – such as government-commissioned recommendations for a separate review body for sexual assault complaints – suggest that the significant self-regulatory powers of the colleges may be beginning to wane.

References

Allsop, J. and Jones, K. (2008) 'Protecting patients: international trends in medical governance', in Kuhlmann, E. and Saks, M. (eds) *Rethinking Professional Governance: International Directions in Healthcare*, Bristol: Policy Press.

Allsop, J. and Saks, M. (eds) (2003) *Regulating the Health Professions*, London: Sage.

Arksey, H. and O'Malley, L. (2005) 'Scoping studies: towards a methodological framework', *International Journal of Social Research Methodology* 8(1): 19-32.

Chamberlain, J. M. (2015) *Medical Regulation, Fitness to Practice and Revalidation: A Critical Introduction*, Bristol: Policy Press.

Cruess, S. R. and Cruess, R. L. (2005) 'The medical profession and self-regulation: a current challenge', *Virtual Mentor* 7(4), http://journalofethics.ama-assn.org/2005/04/oped1-0504.html

Dawson, S. (2013) 'We have no choice but to hire contract doctors, Nunavut's medical boss says', *Nunatsiaq Online*, 15 March.

Deber, R. and Mah, C. (eds) (2014) *Case Studies in Canadian Health Policy and Management* (2nd edition), Toronto: University of Toronto Press.

Dent, M., Chandler, J. and Barry, J. (eds) (2004) *Questioning the New Public Management*, Aldershot: Ashgate.

Donovan, K. (2016) 'Task force calls for independent body to probe alleged sex abuse by doctors', *Toronto Star*, 8 September.

FHRCO (Federation of Health Regulatory Colleges of Ontario) (2015) 'We Care about Your Care', http://www.regulatedhealthprofessions.on.ca/we-care-about-your-care.html

Gallant, J. (2016) 'Refusal to revoke doctor's licence leaves CPSO "disappointed" by its own panel', *Toronto Star*, 28 April.

Horsley, T., Lockyer, J., Cogo, E., Zeiter, J., Bursey, F. and Campbell, C. (2016) 'National programmes for validating physician competence and fitness for practice: a scoping review', *BMJ Open* 6.

Hutchison, B., Levesque, J. F., Strumpf, E. and Coyle, N. (2011) 'Primary health care in Canada: systems in motion', *Milbank Quarterly* 89(2): 256-88.

Institute of Medicine (2001) *Crossing the Quality Chasm: A New Health System for the 21st Century*, Washington, DC: National Academy Press.

Kuhlmann, E. and Saks, M. (2008) 'Changing patterns of health professional governance', in Kuhlmann, E. and Saks, M. (eds) *Rethinking Professional Governance: International Directions in Healthcare*, Bristol: Policy Press.

Levac, D., Colquhoun, H. and O'Brien, K. K. (2010) 'Scoping studies: advancing the methodology', *Implementation Science* 5: 69.

Nadeau, R., Bélanger, E., Pétry, F., Soroka, S. and Maioni, A. (2014) *Health Care Policy and Opinion in the United States and Canada*, New York, NY: Routledge.

Rosenthal, M. (1995) *The Incompetent Doctor: Behind Closed Doors*, Bristol, PA: Open University Press.

Royal College of Physicians and Surgeons of Canada (2016) 'What We Do', Ottawa: Royal College, http://www.royalcollege.ca/rcsite/about/what-we-do-e

Saks, M. (1995) *Professions and the Public Interest: Medical Power, Altruism and Alternative Medicine*, London: Routledge.

Saks, M. (2000) 'Medicine and the counter culture', in Cooter, R. and Pickstone, J. (eds) *Medicine in the 20th Century*, Amsterdam: Harwood Academic Publishers.

Saks, M. (2010) 'Analyzing the professions: the case for a neo-Weberian approach', *Comparative Sociology* 9(6): 887-915.

Saks, M. (2015a) 'Health policy and complementary and alternative medicine', in Kuhlmann, E., Blank, R., Bourgeault, I. and Wendt, C. (eds) *The Palgrave International Handbook of Healthcare Policy and Governance*, Basingstoke: Palgrave Macmillan.

Saks, M. (2015b) *The Professions, State and the Market: Medicine in Britain, the United States and Russia*, Abingdon: Routledge.

Saks, M. (2016) 'Review of theories of professions, organizations and society: neo-Weberianism, neo-institutionalism and eclecticism', *Journal of Professions and Organization* 3(2): 170-87.

Shaw, K., Cassel, C. K., Black, C. and Levinson, W. (2009) 'Shared medical regulation in a time of increasing calls for accountability and transparency: comparison of recertification in the United States, Canada, and the United Kingdom', *Journal of the American Medical Association* 302(18): 2008-14.

Starr, P. (1984) *The Social Transformation of American Medicine*, New York, NY: Basic Books.

Wenghofer, E. F. (2015) 'Research in medical regulation: an active demonstration of accountability', *Journal of Medical Regulation* 101(3): 13-17.

Wenghofer, E. F., Williams, A. P. and Klass, D. J. (2009) 'Factors affecting physician performance: implications for performance management and governance', *Healthcare Policy* 5(2): 141-60.

List of websites

Collège des Médecins du Québec (2016) 'Collège des médecins du Québec', http://www.cmq.org/home.aspx

College of Physicians and Surgeons of Alberta (2016) 'For the Public', http://www.cpsa.ca/public/

College of Physicians and Surgeons of British Columbia (2016) 'Mission, Mandate and Values', https://www.cpsbc.ca/about-us/mission

College of Physicians and Surgeons of Manitoba (2016) 'The Role of the College', http://cpsm.mb.ca/about-the-college/roll-of-the-college

College of Physicians and Surgeons of New Brunswick (2016) 'College of Physicians and Surgeons of New Brunswick - Home', http://cpsnb.org/en/

College of Physicians and Surgeons of Newfoundland and Labrador (2016) 'For the Public', https://www.cpsnl.ca/web/cpsnl

College of Physicians and Surgeons of Nova Scotia (2016) 'CPSNS The College of Physicians and Surgeons of Nova Scotia', https://cpsns.ns.ca/

College of Physicians and Surgeons of Ontario (2016) 'Home College of Physicians and Surgeons of Ontario', http://www.cpso.on.ca/

College of Physicians and Surgeons of Prince Edward Island (2016) 'College of Physicians and Surgeons of Prince Edward Island', http://cpspei.ca/

College of Physicians and Surgeons of Saskatchewan (2016) 'College of Physicians and Surgeons of Saskatchewan (CPSS) Home', https://www.cps.sk.ca/imis/

Department of Health (2016) 'Department of Health Government of Nunavut', https://www.gov.nu.ca/health

FHRCO (Federation of Health Regulatory Colleges of Ontario) (2016) 'We Care about Your Care', http://www.regulatedhealthprofessions.on.ca/we-care-about-your-care.html

Health and Social Services (2016) 'Health and Social Services Promote, Protect, and Provide for the Health and Well-being of the People of the NWT', http://www.hss.gov.nt.ca/

Royal College of Physicians and Surgeons of Canada (2016) 'The Royal College of Physicians and Surgeons of Canada: Home', http://www.royalcollege.ca/rcsite/home-e

Yukon Medical Council (2016) 'Yukon Medical Council - Home Page', http://www.yukonmedicalcouncil.ca/

Let the consumer beware: maintenance of licensure and certification in the United States

Ruth Horowitz

Introduction

Despite news headlines publicising the analysis of data from several large-scale studies by a Johns Hopkins University physician that medical errors (about 250,000 each year) are the third leading cause of death in the United States (US) (Makary and Daniel, 2016), the pushback on requiring continuous education for physicians has been strong. In the US, the public rarely questions whether doctors are keeping up with the latest knowledge and skills. Patients assume that their physicians are up to date and some organisation is keeping track that they are. They are more likely to worry about whether their doctor listens to them (AP and NORC, 2014). Despite the growing interest in the patient safety movement, doctors have few legally embedded requirements to keep up to date in their practice areas. Instead, the mix of players trying to reform requirements is often in conflict and the pushback from multiple sectors to change is strong. This chapter examines the persistent difficulties in ensuring that all physicians keep up with rapidly changing information about diagnoses, treatments and new technological advances.

Ensuring the health and safety of patients in the US requires major resources. In 2014, 916,264 physicians held active licences to practise, a 4% increase from 2012; 207,840 were international medical school graduates and 72,901 were doctors of osteopathy (who have their own medical organisations). Men made up 66% and women 33%. In addition, 78.6% held one state licence, while 15.5% had two and 5.9% had three or more. The percentage of physicians with an active licence holding an American Board of Medical Specialties (ABMS) certification is 79% (Young et al, 2015).

In theory, state medical licensure and specialty board certification provide some continuing competency standards. Decisions about how to ensure competency are made by governmental institutions (state legislatures, federal agencies and state and national courts), a number of market groups (the public, public organisations and insurance companies) and professional organisations (state medical societies, the American Medical Association [AMA], state specialty societies, specialty boards, ABMS and hospitals). The medical licensing and disciplinary boards (each state has at least one) sit differently between the profession and the state government depending on the state medical practice Acts passed by the state legislatures. Their national association is the Federation of State Medical Boards (FSMB). Each state has its own requirements for *licensure* and *licence renewal*. The 'official' 24 specialty boards are medical organisations affiliated with the ABMS and each sets its own requirements for *certification* and *recertification*.

The US extols democratic procedures that bring multiple groups into the debates and market mechanisms that counter state-based regulation. State legislatures created *licensing boards* at the end of the 19th century, which permitted physicians appointed to those boards to license and discipline physicians until the 1960s when public members were first added in California. Today, all but a handful of states include public or consumer representatives on these boards (Horowitz, 2013). Their actions are subject to state and federal judicial review. Since 1965, Medicare (insurance for those aged over 65) and Medicaid (insurance for the very poor) – and in 2010 the Affordable Care Act (ACA), which required all Americans to buy health insurance by 2014 or pay a fine – have allowed more federal involvement. Specialty *certification* is not required for licensure and is controlled by each *specialty board*, which must be recognised by the ABMS. These certification boards are controlled by the medical profession with some recent appointments of public members, but the boards have no legal authority over their membership. Medical organisations, developed over the past hundred years, sometimes operate at cross-purpose as they are propelled by conflicting interests, with little more than persuasion to effect regulatory changes. How, then, does the system ensure that physicians maintain competence over the lifecourse and why is it so difficult to change?

It is possible to leave it to the profession to sort out through Maintenance of Certification (MOC). But this would mean corralling different medical organisations and specialties to improve and standardise specialty board certification requirements. Importantly, about 20% of physicians are not board-certified (FSMB, 2016a). Moreover, many certified before the advent of time-limited certification, largely in the early 1990s, do not have requirements to maintain certification, although those working in hospitals may have some requirements. About two thirds of hospitals require their physicians to be board-certified.

State legislatures can enact new requirements for Maintenance of Licensure (MOL), but this requires cooperation from medical licensing and disciplinary boards and medical organisations (local medical societies and new anti-regulation groups) to refrain from agitating against regulatory changes. Currently, all but five states have continuing medical education (CME) requirements for licence renewal, but only a few require a proportion of credits in the area of practice of the physician. No enforcement mechanism exists to ensure that physicians implement what they learned.

Proposed changes in both MOC and MOL are similar in intent to the revalidation process in Britain (Chamberlain, 2013, 2015). However, the current US regulatory practice leaves major gaps in the standards and their application. Anti-regulation sentiments have been on the rise in the US at national and local levels. The result is that efforts by some medical organisations to nudge others towards greater oversight of their members have been stymied by other medical groups, which have launched legal and political challenges against proposed legislative (MOL) and specialty board recertification (MOC) changes. The very diversity of the institutions with a stake in the regulatory process has complicated the matter. What tends to get lost in this state of affairs is the public interest. The public representation on many boards is rather tenuous, and some physician organisations strongly oppose increased regulation in the name of 'professionalism' and support the free-market approach of many state legislatures.

Licensing in the United States

Before the end of the 19th century when all states enacted licensing statutes, anyone could declare themselves a physician. Legislatures were hesitant to infringe on any person's right to practise medicine (Shryock, 1967). Only after the public health movement began to show that health could be improved in the mid-19th century and the AMA and local societies convinced doctors that licensing would not exclude them, were statutes passed that created state licensing boards with the authority to grant licences at the end of the 19th century. Most states provided several initial pathways to licensure, including having practised in the state for a period of several years (Horowitz, 2013).

The US Supreme Court in *Dent v. West Virginia* (1898) affirmed the right to exclude those who failed to meet a licensing board's criteria from the practise of medicine (Mohr, 1993). By the early 1900s, most states required exams (written by boards) of all graduates of state board-approved medical schools (Johnson and Chaudhry, 2012). The National Board of Medical Examiners (NBME), founded in 1915 by physicians, tried to establish national exams but was only partially successful until the 1970s when all states finally accepted a national exam. Only in the early 1990s did physicians, whether educated abroad or in the US, take the United States Medical Licensing Examination (USMLE) (owned by the FSMB and NBME), with the exception of osteopathic physicians who administer their own.

Most of the state licensing and disciplinary boards members were male physicians until the 1970s when the federal government became interested in the organisation of medicine and cost of health care after the enactment of Medicare and Medicaid. The Department of Labour, concerned that licensing statutes restricted the movement of labour across state lines, thus creating market inefficiencies, and the Department of Health, Education and Welfare, worried about the costs of health care because of medicine's control over the scope of practice that kept nurses and others from doing what they were trained to do at less cost, suggested public members. Local scandals of sexual abuse and terrible health care outcomes played up in the press spurred state legislators to make changes. Nevertheless, three state boards still have no public members (Horowitz, 2013).

Although all state boards currently have approximately the same requirements for licensure, the boards are differently embedded in state bureaucracies – some are run largely by state employees who have substantial decision-making power, and others are largely autonomous from the state and can hire and fire staff, with the board members making a wide range of licensing, discipline and policy decisions. Disciplinary processes and what a physician can be disciplined for vary considerably as does the influence of boards on legislatures. Medical societies (voluntary associations) remain influential in most states. Disciplinary outcomes can be appealed in the state courts.

The FSMB, founded in 1912 as an association of state licensing and disciplinary boards, must rely on persuasion for change. Despite FSMB recommendations that state boards follow, they have achieved little uniformity among the 66 US boards (14 states have separate osteopathic and allopathic boards, New York separates discipline and licensing, and Washington DC has one).

Licensure requires a three-part exam and some years of residency training (variable by state). The only requirements for licence renewal are CME credits – each state has its own number, some mandate particular courses such as pain management or end-of-life decisions, but only a handful require physicians do some percentage in their areas of practice. Five states have no CME requirements. In essence, licensing boards trust physicians to keep up to date in their areas of practice.

Specialty certification

The ABMS is a voluntary association set up by the medical community in 1933 as an 'advisory' board (Stevens, 1998). It currently has 24 specialty boards such as surgery, internal medicine and ophthalmology. These are the only 'recognised' specialty boards, but other groups also claim to certify their members. To obtain certification, each recognised specialty board requires specific advanced training and an exam, but requirements differ.

As medical groups formalised their specialties, they sought formal recognition for those who had the skill and knowledge to do particular tasks. The fight for this system of 'certification' through physician-organised boards was contested at the beginning of the 20th century with various proposals by medical organisations to deal with the growth of specialists and their desire to be recognised as highly trained. Should they have a special diploma or a special licence? The American Association of Medical Colleges wanted graduate education, the NBME wanted to assess and certify, and the Council on Medical Education of the AMA had other ideas. The context was particularly fraught as doctors were not making much money during the Depression and interpreted this failure as an oversupply of physicians. None of the options presented to the specialty boards generated enthusiasm. The AMA was involved but many of the specialty associations developed outside the AMA (Stevens, 1998; Weisz, 2006). However, 70% still identified as general practitioners in 1940 so licensure was the main regulatory mechanism (Rothman, 2003).

The public interest was not discussed (Stevens, 1998), but in the 1930s several specialty associations incorporated boards that specified training requirements and exams. The debates continued over which national group would coordinate the specialty boards and what influence that organisation should have. The main concern was making a living for the physicians, not patient access, cost or safety. By 1940, 14 of the current 24 specialty boards were formed under the auspices of the Advisory Board for Medical Specialties, which did not get along easily with the AMA's Council on Medical Education as the latter was more focused on generalists. It took more than 30 years to change the name to the ABMS, which potentially strengthened its position in the late 1960s (Stevens, 1998). Specialty boards, such as Family Medicine and Internal Medicine, began in the 1970s to enforce time-limited certifications with a recertification exam. But those certified before time-limited licences do not have to meet the new requirements; they are 'grandfathered in'. Hence, a physician could have been certified in 1975, but have done nothing to keep up to date, in five states, unless a hospital requires it.

Although most hospitals require board certification for their staff, that is up to the hospitals in most states. And they may not require it, particularly in rural locations. They may also require CME for staff. Insurance companies do not require certification but some of Medicare health maintenance organisations are beginning to do so. For patients, certification is important; some evidence shows that those who practise medicine without board certification are more likely to have disciplinary actions taken against them than certified physicians (Lipner et al, 2016).

New issues: maintenance of licensure and certification

MOL and MOC have been on the table since 2004 when the FSMB adopted the statement: 'State medical boards have a responsibility to the public to ensure the ongoing competence of physicians seeking re-licensure.' The push for new standards for licence renewal came from the FSMB and for recertification from the ABMS. That is, it arose largely from within the profession. But neither organisation can coerce its membership.

The FSMB, with 185 staff, is funded by ownership with the NBME of the USMLE, which every licensee must pass today. The FSMB has an elected board, working committees, a data bank of disciplined physicians, a data bank that doctors can use to store their credentials to facilitate obtaining licensure in multiple states, model policies on many issues and a journal. Yet, it has only persuasion to entice state boards to support new licence renewal requirements. Several states agreed to serve as models in 2011.

Initially, the FSMB took a strong stand on reformulating what physicians should do for licence renewal, but new requirements would entail changes in each state; many would need legislation. The MOL framework would entail:

- 'reflective self-assessment' and the requirement that the majority of CME credits be practice-relevant;
- assessment of knowledge and skills;
- assessment of performance.

The FSMB argued for a slow and phased entry, participation in MOC counting for MOL, and consistency of MOL requirements across states to facilitate maintaining multiple licences (FSMB, 2015b).

After reformulating model requirements for recertification, the ABMS created a working committee (Committee on Continuing Certification or 3C) made up of representatives from each specialty board and two public members to use the new standards to access specialty board changes in requirements to ensure some consistency among the boards while maintaining flexibility and relevance. These standards, developed in 2012-13, involved contributions from the public, member boards, the ABMS board of directors, several ABMS committees, specialty societies, diplomates and associate member organisations. The intent was to emphasise a model of continuing development – both learning and assessment to align with other quality improvements and educational and regulatory activities in which physicians were already engaging.

Six core competencies were adopted in 1999:

- practice-based learning and improvement;
- patient care and procedural skills;
- systems-based practice;
- medical knowledge;
- interpersonal and communications skills;
- professionalism.

These are to be integrated in the four parts of the MOC:

- professionalism;
- lifelong learning and self-assessment (mostly continuing education);
- assessment of knowledge, judgement and skills;
- improvement of medical practice.

All new certifications are time-limited, but new rules do not cover those who were 'grandfathered in' or the physicians who are not board-certified. Additionally, physicians who are board-certified and do not practise in a hospital that requires specialty certification could let it lapse, probably with little consequence to their income as most members of the public do not ask. Both the FSMB and ABMS have used 'the public interest' to frame their discussion of changes; nevertheless, a discussion of the public interest does not appear in the discussions of many physicians' organisations and state legislatures.

Legislature pushback

Some state legislatures favour a market-oriented approach. They may worry about having a sufficient number of physicians or have been encouraged by local medical societies to maintain things as they are. About 11 states have initiated legislative Bills that would not permit changes to licence renewal or, in some cases, are prohibiting requiring certification for practice in institutions.

This legislation obstructs both MOL and MOC changes and is based, whether intended or not, on a theory that the market is strong enough to ensure that patients can assess and pick physicians without much information. It assumes that, as professionals, physicians are keeping their practices current. Two such Bills are the following:

> Nothing in the Oklahoma Allopathic Medical and Surgical Licensure and Supervision Act shall be construed as to require a physician to secure a Maintenance of Certification (MOC) as a condition of licensure, reimbursement, employment or admitting privileges at a hospital in this state. For the purposes of this subsection, 'Maintenance of Certification (MOC)' shall mean a continuing education program measuring core competencies in the practice of medicine and surgery and approved by a nationally recognized accrediting organization. (Oklahoma SB 1148 2016)
>
> The board shall not require any form of maintenance of licensure as a condition of physician licensure, including requiring any form of maintenance of licensure tied to maintenance of certification. The board's regular requirements, including continuing medical education, shall suffice to demonstrate professional competency.
>
> ... The board shall not require any form of specialty medical board certification or any maintenance of certification to practice medicine in Kentucky.' (Kentucky SB 17 2016)

Let the buyer beware is the implication of these legislative Bills. Patients should leave it to the individual physician to ensure safety.

Local and national medical organisations push back against change

The likelihood that state legislatures moved to block changes on their own initiative was small. State medical societies generally instigated the legislation. Moreover, the American Association of Physicians and Surgeons (AAPS), a small group of anti-regulation physicians who founded their association in 1943 and call themselves 'private' physicians, filed a law suit on 23 April 2013 against the ABMS for restraint of trade and reducing the number of doctors by its onerous and expensive criteria for recertification, without improving the quality of patient care. This scared the FSMB and the ABMS. The case, filed in New Jersey, argued that a doctor trying to serve people living in poverty could not afford to be recertified. The petitioners partially relied on their survey, answered by only 185 doctors, who thought that recertification was a waste (AAPS, 2012). The brief claimed:

> Members of Plaintiff AAPS have suffered injury in the form of thousands of dollars of unjustified expense, hundreds of hours taken away from their care of patients, the exclusion from hospital medical staffs, and reputational harm, all due to the conduct and statements by Defendant ABMS as alleged herein. Plaintiff's requested declaratory and injunctive relief will prevent ongoing and imminent future injury. The protection of AAPS members from the antitrust violations and misrepresentations alleged herein is central to AAPS's purpose of safeguarding the practice of private medicine against interference. (Civil Action, No. 3:13-cv-2609-PGS-LHG: 4)

A 'White Paper' by the group's president is critical of the FSMB for proposing to expand criteria for licence renewal. The FSMB writes:

> [I]n virtually all states, it is possible for a physician to practice medicine for a lifetime without having to demonstrate to the state medical board that he or she has maintained an acceptable level of continuing qualifications or competence. Citing rapid advances in science and technology, the FSMB thinks this leniency is no longer acceptable, and has drafted

a 58-page report that was submitted for comments due in January 2008. Unnoticed by most state licensure boards and medical organizations, the effort by the FSMB to subject physicians to increasingly intrusive regulation has been going on for some time, with the support of the American Association of Retired Persons (AARP), the American Medical Association (AMA), Blue Cross/Blue Shield Association, and the Robert Wood Johnson Foundation. The 'guidance' for the 'core competencies' that physicians would have to demonstrate.... (Orient, 2008: 23)

This statement was written by Jane M. Orient, M.D., F.A.C.P., executive director of AAPS and an internist. Licensing boards knew about this FSMB report as it was written by FSMB board members and discussed at annual FSMB meetings. The following statement was posted on the AAPS website dated 5 November 2015:

By the FSMB's definition, the instant you stop participating in proprietary, costly MOC, or fail an exam, *you are no longer a physician! MOC means that you are no longer a professional, but a subordinate of self-appointed higher authorities.* You will be constantly on probation, subject to a never-ending round of examinations that may be completely unrelated to what you do every day. *AAPS, unlike most medical associations, has been fighting this monster.* (AAPS, 2015)

A more moderate critic wrote:

There has been a significant amount of outrage over the past few months of the maintenance of certification process. The anger has not only been targeted towards the ABIM [American Board of Internal Medicine], but also towards the other specialty boards. Pediatrics, for example, now requires ABP approved quality improvement (QI) projects that have been widely criticized. While these MOC requirements are a major nuisance for most, the implications may actually run much deeper. A number of doctors are opting out of medicine and citing increasing maintenance of certification requirements as a major contributing factor. (Paul, 2016)

Letters appeared on internet sites criticising MOC:

> Wow. For those who think MOC isn't a big deal, my open letter to the American Board of Pediatrics just hit 70,000 views. That's stunning. For those commending my bravery, realize efforts like this are not done in isolation … I also have the support of my state medical society. Michigan State Medical Society has the strongest state policy on MOC in the country: MOC should not be tied to licensure, hospital privileges or insurance participation and it should not be the monopoly of one organization. It helps knowing there's a 15,000 member society on my side…. If you think you need MOC to practice, please make sure. Check your insurance contracts. Check your hospital privileges. (Edison, 2016)

With 'self-regulation', any new group can set itself up to 'certify' physicians. Moreover, with some of the new state legislation, it may encourage hospitals to not require board certification of doctors on staff. Thus, patients may have little information on current knowledge and skills when choosing or being cared for by a physician and may be treated by doctors who have not kept up to date.

Where is the public?

Licensure is not an area that inspires high non-physician activism, though a particular issue or disciplinary case may catch a group's attention, particularly when a friend or family member is seen as suffering in the hands of a problematic physician. Consumer and patient groups are not as well organised as the profession and most are local and narrowly focused.

The Consumers Union, which has a long history of evaluating and rating consumer goods such as cars and washing machines, has turned in the past decade to issues affecting health. It takes a market-based approach, working to make patients better consumers by expanding access to data with information on hospitals and doctors. This has been an approach taken by some consumer groups since the 1960s (Tomes, 2015). They have been pushing a Bill in California, for example, to require physicians on probation by the licensing board to alert their patients so that the patients can make informed decisions about whether to find new physicians. The Consumers Union has collected 6,000 stories of people who say they were harmed by medical errors and formed the Patient Safety Action Network, which is pushing for medical board transparency and other consumer and safety issues. Much of the focus is to improve the patient's position in the marketplace (McGiffert, 2016). Sidney Wolfe's *Public Citizen* (an organisation related to Ralph Nader's group) has ranked state boards by the percentage of disciplined doctors and rated medical board websites for the information they have provided.

The public is interested in getting more and improved information about their doctors, but for now, they turn mostly to friends and family to find health care providers and evaluate them. What people say they want from their providers is a doctor who can communicate well with them, one who listens and seems to care, according to recent survey data (AP and NORC, 2014). The public assumes that mechanisms are in place to keep doctors' skills and knowledge current. Although public members do sit on many of the boards and press public protection, few citizens know much about regulation, despite stories of regulatory failure in the press and the availability of disciplinary and specialty data on 'Docinfo' on the FSMB website (Horowitz, 2013).

The judiciary raises new issues

Public complaints as expressed in local presses' stories are frequent in many states and can influence legislatures, but the courts have considerable authority over licensing and disciplinary boards. All disciplinary cases can be appealed, but more important is the US Supreme Court's opinion in *North Carolina Board of Dental Examiners v. FTC* (Federal Trade Commission) on 25 February 2015, which has shaken up boards of many licenced occupations. The FSMB and the AMA supplied Amicus briefs, briefs submitted with supplemental information to the appellate courts, on behalf of the Dental Board. In the North Carolina case, the board's anti-competitive action that caused the FTC to intervene was writing cease-and-desist letters to non-dentists doing teeth whitening, threatening criminal liability if they continued to provide whitening services. The dental board made no mention of patient harm.

The court found in favour of the FTC's position that a licensing board controlled by 'active market participants' (a term not defined in the court's opinion) cannot invoke the state action antitrust immunity unless the board was subject to 'active supervision by the state'. The Supreme Court ruled that the board could not be granted immunity from prosecution as a state agency as the state had little supervision over its work. The court rejected the contention raised by the dental board and by several occupational licensing boards and their federations that the FTC order would discourage dedicated citizens from serving on regulatory boards. In reaction to the court, 11 states have developed new legislation to increase state purview over the scope of practice issues or provided statements affirming board immunity from liability under state and federal antitrust laws.

The language used by the Supreme Court in their opinion was that of the market-based economy: 'Federal antitrust law is a central safeguard for the Nation's free market structure.' It does not mean that the states cannot place restrictions on occupations that allow them to control the market and limit competition, but it is within the court's power to sit in judgement on whether they have gone too far – that is, whether 'active market participants' are in charge (not the state) and private anti-competitive motives might be in play.

Results of pushback: the Interstate Compact as a substitute

With the pushback from local medical societies and legislators, the legal cases, and general lack of support, the FSMB no longer discusses licence renewal. It last appeared in about 2012 as a topic for discussion at the annual meetings when several states expressed interest in adopting new standards. Some interest remains within the organisation, however, and it continues to do some research on what doctors are doing to maintain their professional development (FSMB, 2015b).

Instead, the FSMB is focusing on the Interstate Compact, which will facilitate holding multiple licences and the practice of telemedicine. It may also aid in forestalling a national licensure movement. The Interstate Compact is a contract between states, which, according to the FSMB, will increase access to care through facilitating physicians' obtaining licences in multiple states without the loss of state authority to discipline (FSMB, 2015a). It will allow physicians, holding a time-limited specialty certification by an ABMS-approved board, to apply for multiple licences without having to go through the entire licensing procedure. Sessions at the FSMB annual meeting focus on the Interstate Compact and efforts to coordinate state licensing processes have been successful, as the following press release demonstrates:

> WASHINGTON, D.C. (January 21, 2016) – Kicking off the 2016 state legislative season, six new states have introduced legislation to enact the Interstate Medical Licensure Compact.... Twelve states have enacted the Compact ... which offers a streamlined licensing process for physicians interested in practicing medicine in multiple states, is expected to expand access to health care, especially

to those in rural and underserved areas of the country, and facilitate new modes of health care delivery such as telemedicine. Thirty-one state medical and osteopathic boards have publicly expressed support for the Compact, and it has been endorsed by a broad coalition of health care stakeholders, including the American Medical Association (AMA) and the American Osteopathic Association (AOA). (FSMB, 2016b)

Additional states joined after this press release.

Not all physicians buy in to the new process, however. They want to limit the market, but they do not want the system or rules that come with state market limitations. The AAPS is pushing back and contested the efforts to coordinate state licensing processes: 'Help STOP the FSMB from continuing its efforts to bury physicians in red tape.' On 31 January 2015, a letter posted on its website was entitled: 'FSMB insults physicians and patients with attempt to defend power grab' (AAPS, 2015). The ABMS, in the meantime, is dealing with efforts by some of its larger boards to stop changes in the recertification process. ABMS continues to push change, but the pushback is strong.

Federal government's efforts at education and demonstrating competency: opioids and the Medicare Access and CHIP Reauthorization Act 2015

The increased costs of Medicare and a series of deaths of middle-class young people following abuse of physician-prescribed medications have led to calls for more involvement of the federal government in the regulation of prescribing. In 2014, about 19,000 deaths resulted from opioid pain relievers and over 8,000 deaths from benzodiazepines, a greater number than deaths from cocaine and heroin (National Institute on Drug Abuse, 2017). First, the *New York Times* reported in 2016 that the federal government (under President Obama) proposed to require doctors who prescribe opioids to have training. Second, the increasing cost of Medicare led to changes in reimbursements requiring an assessment of the value of care under the Medicare Access and CHIP Reauthorization Act (MACRA), which was signed into law on 16 April 2015.

The uncontrolled use of pain medications has created problems of abuse. The first criminal case against a physician for second-degree murder for the fatal overdoses of three young males in their twenties was successfully prosecuted in a Californian trial lasting eight weeks, with the jury deliberating for two additional weeks. As the *Los Angeles Times* documented, the case was complicated with 77 witnesses and 250 pieces of evidence. Despite the overwhelming evidence of arrests of 'pill mill' doctors who sell opioids to 'patients', and the enormous caseloads of state medical boards dealing with opioid prescribing, doctors are fighting federal educational requirements.

When a Federal Drug Administration (FDA) panel recommended that opioid prescribers take a mandatory training course, it was rejected. The *New York Times* noted in 2016:

> At first, Dr. Katz, who had been on the panel, thought that drug makers had pressured the F.D.A. to kill the proposal. Then an agency official told him that another group had fought the recommendation: the American Medical Association, the nation's largest physician organization. 'I was shocked,' said Dr. Katz.... (Meier, 2016)

Not only is the AMA against mandatory training, it is also opposed to laws that require doctors to check databases that might slow drug-seeking behaviour. The AMA does not represent all physicians as it has only 217,000 members of almost one million licenced physicians. Some state medical societies are working to limit the use of painkillers, but many doctors have little training in their use.

Some states are addressing overprescribing. Kentucky, hard hit by high rates of opioid addiction, in 2012 began to require that physicians and other prescribers check patients in the drug database before prescribing in order to determine whether patients were receiving prescriptions from multiple sources. Fifteen other states did the same and 29 require checking under certain conditions. Evidence shows that the law requiring physicians to check the database has some effect. In Kentucky, opioid use dropped very significantly between 2012 and 2013, the first year the law was implemented, according to a study by the University of Kentucky's College of Pharmacy (Freeman et al, 2015).

But Missouri did not want a database. The creation of a prescription drug monitoring system in Missouri has been blocked by a small group of legislators, led by state Senator Rob Schaaf, a Republican and physician, who filibustered a Bill that would allow the government to keep prescription records because it would violate patient privacy rights and if 'they overdose and kill themselves, it just removes them from the gene pool' (Skolek, 2012).

MACRA involves a new payment system for physicians serving Medicare recipients (all those who are at least 65 are eligible for Medicare insurance, for which all earners are taxed). The new payment scheme is intended to modify the traditional 'fee for service' model and includes measures of quality to determine the fee received by physicians. What that quality is or how it should be measured is still debated. Statements from a number of sources claim that no sufficient quality measures exist; therefore, physicians should not have their fees determined by 'quality' measures. The AMA wishes to hold onto the current payment system of customary and reasonable fees.

The new payment system, the 'Merit-based Incentive Payment System' (MIPS), begins in 2019, the incentives for which will be based on the quality of care (30%), resource use (30%), meaningful use of electronic medical records (25%) and clinical improvement activities (15%). The last one is similar to Part IV of the ABMS board recertification model. Some argue that the system will use performance metrics, surveys of patient experience and outcome measures (Oberlander and Laugesen, 2015).

Some medical groups opposing MOL and MOC are also opposed to the new Medicare plans:

> The Association of American Physicians and Surgeons, AAPS, has been fighting the good fight to preserve the practice of private medicine since 1943. When the Clinton health plan was proposed, we fought for open meetings. And when the details came to light, the plan was halted. In the current battle over health care 'reform,' the AAPS helped organize numerous physician rallys and has a pending lawsuit in the DC Federal District Court challenging the constitutionality of the ObamaCare insurance mandate.... The AAPS seminar, 'Thrive Don't Just Survive', has reached doctors all over the country who wish to leave the hassles of Medicare and the interference of managed care and start a cash practice. We have helped hundreds of doctors opt out of Medicare through information on our website and our limited legal consultation service. (AAPS, 2015)

How much influence this organisation or the AMA will have is open to question as medicine does not speak with one voice. But it is difficult to know how much influence these organisations will have, especially when licensing and specialty boards take different positions.

Conclusion: regulating care in a market-based democracy

Democracies have different ways of regulating health care providers, organising health care, and providing health care insurance. The US is traditionally anti-regulation; some are against it even when their group is doing the regulating and others perhaps because the US has regulated so many occupations. It is also a consumerist culture. After medicine obtained licensure and could control access to the profession, it created its own regulatory organisations (exam, hospital and specialty organisations). Only the addition of public members provides another voice in regulation with a few limits from courts and legislatures. Nevertheless, the profession remains the strongest force in determining 'the public interest'.

Given the US culture and local systems, the conflicts over revalidation in Britain look quite straightforward. The British NHS may need to 'bring doctors along', but it is one government organisation that pays for all medical care and the General Medical Council is one organisation that regulates all practising physicians. In the US, some professional organisations claim to be working on behalf of 'the public interest' and see a need to ensure continuing competency, but are faced with strong resistance from other medical organisations and physicians and from state legislatures. There resistance not only to 'high stakes exams' but also to any changes at all. Revalidation has avoided the high stakes exam issue by focusing on patient and peer evaluations, a softer approach. Additionally, specialists who have lifetime certificates make the argument of the need to improve recertification to protect the public interest more difficult as those specialists need do little except what the states require for relicensure (very little and in five states almost nothing).

The pressures for market-oriented and anti-big government solutions work with professionalism and self-regulation to stymie regulatory changes. When some medical organisations have asked physicians to demonstrate that they are current in their practices, expressing the reasons as patient safety and improved care, other physician groups take action against change with the support of state legislatures. When the federal government attempts to say that physicians need to take an opioid prescribing course because of the high rates of deaths from opioid abuse or to demonstrate that they are providing good health care, the uproar deters the possibility of change. Despite the International Association of Medical Regulatory Authorities resolution on 22 September 2016 to improve the quality and safety of patient care through developing continuing competency practices, the practicalities of real change on the ground are more significant in determining what happens. As voluntary agencies and as linked to state legislatures, medical organisations have few teeth to tighten regulations in the US.

With the separation of powers engrained in a democratic polity and federal system valorising state autonomy, the potential for conflict and interminable delays in decision making is great. In a country favouring the market and sympathetic to a libertarian ideology, it is difficult to increase regulations upholding the public interest. Lacking strong organisations, patients' interests are bound to suffer in the internecine battles over regulation. The ABMS and FSMB often invoke 'patient safety' and the 'interests of patients' to justify their positions of increased regulation, but they do not speak for the AMA, the local medical societies, or groups of physicians who oppose new requirements. State legislators in many states do not feel that the government should be in the business of regulation so they are primed when the local medical society argues that changing licence renewal requirements is too burdensome. These medical organisations and state legislatures appear to ignore that patients are harmed or die, receive unnecessary treatment or are harmed by medical errors by doctors who do not keep up to date.

Physicians seem to have it both ways – only a little information is available to make better consumers of patients so the market cannot work well (let alone insurance restrictions on physician choice) and physicians have been quite successful at limiting regulatory changes to demonstrate continuing competency. In the current regulatory climate, the prospects for systematic change remain limited. Even if ABMS boards are able to change the recertification process and a few drop certification, more than 20% of practising physicians are not certified and others have lifetime certificates.

Acknowledgement

I would like to thank David Johnson, Frances Cain, Dmitri Shalin and John Martyn Chamberlain for their helpful comments on this chapter.

References

AAPS (Association of American Physicians and Surgeons) (2012) *Survey*, Tucson, AZ: AAPS, https://aapaonline.org/moc-survey-summ/

AAPS (2015) *Report*, Tucson, AZ: AAPS.

AP and NORC (Associated Press and National Opinion Research Center) (2014) *Finding Quality Doctors: How Americans Find Quality Doctors in the U.S.: Research Report*, New York, NY: AP and NORC.

Chamberlain, J. M. (2013) *The Sociology of Medical Regulation: An Introduction*, London: Springer.

Chamberlain, J. M. (2015) *Medical Regulation, Fitness to Practise and Revalidation*, Bristol: Policy Press.

Civil Action, No. 3:13-cv-2609-PGS-LHG in United States District Court for the District of New Jersey, www.aapsonline.org/AAPSvABMScomplaint.pdf

Edison, M. (2016) 'You say you want a revolution', Rebel.MD, 18 January, http://rebel.md/you-say-you-want-a-revolution

FSMB (Federation of State Medical Boards) (2015a) *Inter-State Medical Licensing Compact*, Euless, TX: FSMB.

FSMB (2015b) *Annual Report*, Euless, TX: FSMB

FSMB (2016a) *US Medical Regulatory Trends and Actions*, Euless, TX: FSMB.

FSMB (2016b) 'Six new states introduce interstate medical licensure compact legislation', press release, 21 January.

Horowitz, R. (2013) *In the Public Interest, Medical Licensing and the Disciplinary Process*, New Brunswick, NJ: Rutgers University Press.

Johnson, D. and Chaudhry, H. (2012) *Medical Licensing and Discipline in America*, Lexington, MA: Lexington Books.

Kentucky SB 17 (2016) An Act relating to physicians signed by the governor on 8 April 2016, www.lrc.ky.gov/record/16rs/SB17.htm

Lipner, R., Young, A., Chaudhry, H., Duhigg, L. and Papadakis, M. (2016) 'Specialty certification status, performance ratings, and disciplinary actions of internal medicine residents', *Academic Medicine* 91(3): 376-81.

Makary, M. and Daniel, M. (2016) 'Medical error – the third leading cause of death in the US', *British Medical Journal* 353(2139): 2140.

Meier, B. (2016) 'Opioid prescribing gets another look as F.D.A. revisits mandatory doctor training', *The New York Times*, 2 May, https://www.nytimes.com/2016/05/03/business/fda-again-reviews-mandatory-training-for-painkiller-prescribers.html?_r=0

Mohr, J. (1993) *Doctors and the Law*, Baltimore, MD: Johns Hopkins University Press.

National Institute on Drug Abuse (2017) 'Overdose death rates', https://www.drugabuse.gov/related-topics/trends-statistics/overdose-death-rates

Oberlander, J. and Laugesen, M. (2015) 'Leap of faith – Medicare's new physician payment system', *New England Journal of Medicine* 373: 1185-7.

Oklahoma SB 1148 (2016) An Act signed by the Senate on 1 March and the House on 4 April, http://webserver1.lsb.state.ok.us/cf_pdf/2015-16%20ENR/SB/SB1148%20ENR.PDF

Orient, J. (2008) 'White Paper in opposition to Federation of State Medical Boards (FSMB) proposal on maintenance of licensure', *Journal of American Physicians and Surgeons* 13(1): 23-6, www.jpands.org/vol13no1/orient.pdf

Paul, A. (2016) 'Want to fix MOC? This is one idea to do it', Kevin.MD.com, www.kevinmd.com/blog/2016/04/want-fix-moc-one-idea.html

Rothman, D. (2003) *Strangers at the Bedside*, New York, NY: Aldine.

Shryock, R. (1967) *Medical Licensing in America 1650-1965*, Baltimore, MD: Johns Hopkins University Press.

Skolek, M. (2012) 'There's a conflict of interest on Flamingo Road but no shortage of traffic!', Salem-News.com, www.salem-news.com/articles/october142012/flamingo-road-ms.php

Stevens, R. (1998) *American Medicine in the Public Interest*, Berkeley, CA: University of California Press.

Tomes, N. (2015) *Remaking of the American Patient*, New York, NY: Oxford University Press.

Weisz, G. (2006) *Divide and Conquer*, New York, NY: Oxford University Press.

Young, A., Chaudhry, H., Pei, X., Halbesleben, K., Polk, D. and Dugan, M. (2015) 'A census of actively licensed physicians in the US 2014', *Journal of Medical Regulation* 101(2): 7-23.

TEN

Governing complementary and alternative medicine (CAM) in Brazil and Portugal: implications for CAM professionals and the public

Joana Almeida, Pâmela Siegel and Nelson Barros

Introduction

Since the 'revival' of complementary and alternative medicine (CAM) in the wake of the counterculture of the 1960s/1970s in Western societies (Cant and Sharma, 1999; Saks, 2015a), the issue of the governance of CAM has become a key area for sociological research. The continual acceptance of and/or contestation over CAM treatments and practices by multiple social actors have become too important to be dismissed. In this chapter, the term CAM governance is used thus in a broad sense to designate the various ways in which key actors have regulated CAM. Among these are:

- the state and its different institutions;
- supra–state agencies such as the World Health Organization (WHO);
- professional bodies, CAM practitioners, medical doctors and other allied health care professionals;
- health care corporations such as health insurance companies;
- the lay public.

All have performed a key role in current CAM policy making in many Western countries.

Although sociological research on CAM governance has significantly increased, it remains mainly focused on single countries, rarely being compared internationally. Brazil and Portugal are two helpful examples to compare, for despite their close historical, political and cultural relations, which have spanned centuries, and although there are similarities in their health systems, they present differences in the way they have governed CAM. In this chapter, we compare recent modes of CAM governance in these two distinct yet historically, politically and culturally related countries. We investigate:

- the extent to which CAM governance has changed over the past decades in the two countries;
- the main modes of CAM governance in these same countries;
- the implications of these modes of CAM governance for CAM professionals and for the public.

This chapter is based on a qualitative analysis of legislative and policy documents related to CAM in Brazil and Portugal since the late 1980s. The chapter first offers some theoretical reflections on the complexity of governing CAM in contemporary Western societies. It then analyses CAM's main modes of governance, focusing first on Brazil and then on Portugal. In both cases, the implications of CAM governance for CAM professionals and for the public are addressed. Finally, in the conclusion, CAM's recent modes of governance in Brazil and in Portugal and their implications for CAM professionals and the public are put into comparative perspective.

Governing complementary and alternative medicine: a complex phenomenon

The multiple actors involved in CAM governance in Western societies have made the latter a complex phenomenon. For example, although the WHO has encouraged some degree of harmonisation in developing legislation for traditional and complementary medicine across countries, it has at the same time given freedom to each individual state to regulate CAM (Wiesener et al, 2012). As a result, state governance of CAM has embodied diverse patterns, not only at the national level, varying considerably from country to country, but also within each country, with legislation varying according to the CAM therapies concerned. In countries such as the United Kingdom (UK), for instance, osteopathy and chiropractic have been statutorily regulated since 1993 and 1994 respectively (Saks, 2015b), and therefore achieved state social closure (Parkin, 1979). Yet some other CAM therapies such as acupuncture and homeopathy have developed voluntary self-regulated bodies with registers accredited by the Professional Standards Authority for Health and Social Care, which now governs such practices (Saks, 2015a).

Within the sociology of professions, this multifaceted regulatory framework for CAM in the UK illustrates the coexistence of and the contrast between different styles of professionalism, or ways of organising work and controlling workers. First, CAM regulation in the UK has shown elements of what Evetts (2011) regards as 'organisational professionalism' – a professionalism that has been imposed from 'above', where CAM practitioners have been controlled by forces external to their occupational group such as the state, and where notions of bureaucracy, standardisation, assessment and performance reviews have tended to prevail. Such has been the case for osteopathy and chiropractic, which have been situated at a point on the state exclusionary closure spectrum. Second, CAM regulation in the UK has also led to a professionalism practised from 'within' the occupational group, an 'occupational professionalism', where voluntary self-regulated CAM practitioners have had the freedom to organise and control their work, and where notions of collegiality, discretion and trust have tended to dominate (Evetts, 2011). Such has been the case with acupuncture and homeopathy, which lie at a point on the scale of voluntary self-regulation.

Furthermore, CAM regulation has usually been difficult to analyse as many countries have statutory regulation for CAM treatments and therapies, but not for CAM professions – that is, autonomous and independent occupational groups with legal monopolies recognised by the state (Saks, 2012). This is the case for homeopathic treatments/therapies in 22 countries in Europe, according to 2012 data from the CAMbrella project (Wiesener et al, 2012). In these countries, the profession of the traditional homeopath is not statutorily regulated, although other conventional health care professionals such as medical doctors can provide homeopathic treatments.

Moreover, in countries such as Australia, Canada (Ontario) and the United States (US), governments have regulated therapies such as acupuncture as both a profession and a therapy. For example, in 2013 in Ontario, Canada, traditional Chinese medicine practitioners who have been granted statutory regulation together with chiropractors, naturopaths and homeopaths, and nine biomedically trained professions, were authorised to use acupuncture in their practice (Ijaz et al, 2016). This mode of governance therefore combines an indigenous with a biomedical epistemic framework: if in one case it protects traditional medical knowledge, in another it divorces acupuncture from its traditional framework of Chinese medicine, leading to its medicalisation (Conrad, 2007), incorporation (Saks, 1995) or co-optation (Baer and Coulter, 2008) and therefore cultural 'misappropriation' (Ijaz et al, 2016).

In addition, if different modes of CAM governance and provision within health care have been a main concern for contemporary sociological research, modes of CAM governance and provision within higher education institutions have received comparatively less attention, although their frequency is on the rise. Givati (2015) and Givati and Hatton (2015), for example, have highlighted a number of significant challenges to the formalisation and standardisation of acupuncture education in the UK, including the diverse nature of acupuncture theory, making it too difficult to standardise and codify, and the attacks from some scientists and academics outside CAM circles who actively oppose the teaching of 'academic acupuncture' within higher education institutions, claiming that it is unscientific and non-academic. Brosnan (2015, 2016) has also shown the same epistemological conflict in Australian universities, a conflict that is not very different from that of the health care field as a whole.

To conclude, these examples of CAM governance within health care and higher education across and within countries and continents illustrate:

- the diversity of the CAM field in terms of its relationship with the state and conventional health care professionals, its diverse modalities, philosophical basis and organisational structure;
- the coexistence of different forms of regulation, from voluntary self-regulation to full state closure.

In the next section we show how CAM has been governed in Brazil.

CAM governance in Brazil

Brazil has been a federal presidential constitutional republic since 1889, currently consisting of 26 states and one federal district, each with their own legislation and governor. As a former Portuguese colony, the country evolved to an independent nation during the first half of the 19th century. From 1930 to 1945, Brazil was under Getúlio Vargas' fascist regime, and from 1964 to 1985, the country lived under a military dictatorship, which controlled the government. Since then, a new republic has been established, with the aim of re-establishing democracy, and in 1988 a new federal constitution was adopted (Burns, 1993).

The Brazilian Unified Health System (*Sistema Único de Saúde*, SUS) was born out of the sanitary reform promoted in the 1970s, under and against the military dictatorship, and was inspired by the Italian

Riforma Sanitaria, which created the *Istituzione del Servizio Sanitario Nazionale* in 1978 (Bahia, 2009). The SUS was established by the 1988 federal constitution, which recognised health as a duty of the state and a citizen's right. It is based on the principles of universality, integrality and social participation and was driven by civil society (Chamber of Deputies Directing Board, 2010). The SUS is tailored to cover health promotion, surveillance and education, is financed at the federal, state and municipal levels and includes primary, secondary, tertiary and hospital care. However, due to competing state-supported health care services in the private sector, the SUS is still struggling to achieve universal coverage, although it has greatly improved access to primary and emergency care, vaccination and prenatal coverage, and essential pharmaceutical production (Paim et al, 2011). The National Council of Health (*Conselho Nacional de Saúde*) is the organisation that supervises and governs health care in the country.

State governance of CAM in the country also started in the 1980s, particularly after the foundation of the SUS. Such state interest was inspired by the Declaration of Alma-Ata, adopted at the International Conference of Primary Healthcare held in the former USSR in 1978, where the WHO promoted an integrative, multiprofessional strategy for national health care systems (WHO, 1978). From the 1980s to 2003, therefore, many attempts were made by Brazilian state agencies to govern the inclusion of CAM therapies in the SUS. Some examples were a 1985 agreement between the National Institute for Medical Assistance and Social Security, the State University of Rio de Janeiro, the public health Foundation Oswaldo Cruz and the Brazilian Hahnemannian Institute, with the intention of including homeopathic assistance in the public health sector; a 1999 document (Ministry of Health of Brazil, 1999) decreeing inclusion of medical homeopathy and acupuncture consultations in the list of procedures of SUS; and the various national health conferences held since the 1980s recommending the inclusion of CAM therapies, such as acupuncture, homeopathy, phytotherapy and thermalism, in primary care.

In 2003, during ex-President Lula da Silva's governance, the Department of Primary Care set up a working group made up of representatives from the Science, Technology and Strategic Inputs Secretariat, the Health Work and Education Management Secretariat, the National Health Inspection Agency and the national associations of homeopathy, acupuncture, phytotherapy and anthroposophical medicine, to discuss and prepare a national policy document recommending the inclusion of 'natural medicine and complementary practices' within the SUS (Ministry of Health of Brazil, 2008). As a result, four subgroups were created, and in 2003 an action plan was drafted. Nationwide forums were held, with the extensive participation of civil society organisations, as well as technical meetings to systematise the action plan. An assessment of CAM status at the state and municipal health care levels was conducted by the Department of Primary Care, including a survey carried out from March to June 2004 of all state and municipal health system managers (totalling 5,560), on such features as the installed capacity, the number and profile of professionals involved, the training of human resources and the quality of services. The findings from the questionnaires returned (24% response rate) showed the use of CAM therapies in 232 municipalities, including 19 state capitals, in 26 states in total (Ministry of Health of Brazil, 2008).

In December 2005, the proposed National Policy on Natural Medicine and Complementary Practices was approved by the National Council of Health (CNS), with reservations expressed on the content of the technical autonomy for traditional Chinese medicine/acupuncture and the name of the policy. The council recommended a revision of the text for traditional Chinese medicine/acupuncture, as well as the inclusion of social thermalism and crenotherapy in the policy, based on the results of a report of the Water Group of the CNS (Ministry of Health of Brazil, 2008). In February 2006, after full approval by the CNS, the policy document was finalised, and subsequently published in May under Act 971. Act 971 sanctions the National Policy for Integrative and Complementary Practices (PNPIC) (note the change of terms), and allows for homeopathy, traditional Chinese medicine/acupuncture, phytotherapy and social thermalism/crenotherapy to be practised within the SUS.

In July 2006, however, Act 1600 was published, sanctioning the request from the Brazilian Association of Anthroposophical Medicine to create an Observatory of Anthroposophical Medicine within the SUS, thus adding this therapy to the list of therapies approved by Act 971 (Ministry of Health of Brazil, 2006). Briefly, it can be stated that the development of the PNPIC in the SUS followed recommendations from different national health bodies over the years, and was encouraged by the SUS's principles of universality, integrality and social participation – as well as by the WHO strategy for traditional medicine from 2002 to 2005, which recommended the implementation of CAM policies, taking into special consideration its security, efficacy, quality, use and access (WHO, 2002).

Although the PNPIC was designed to include a limited number of CAM practices at a multiprofessional level in the Family Health Strategy of Primary Care, homeopathy, acupuncture and anthroposophical medicine have become medical specialties within the SUS. Homeopathy, which was officially introduced in Brazil in 1840, had been already recognised as a medical specialty in 1980 (Monteiro and Iriart, 2007). Yet Salles (2008) shows its weak presence in Brazilian medical faculties, with 35 out of 115 medical colleges not offering any homeopathic-related content in their medical courses, and only 17 out of 115 doing it, in 2005. Furthermore, most of these colleges either promoted homeopathy as a minor discipline or offered homeopathic-related content in other disciplines (Salles, 2008). De Barros and Fiuza (2014) have also highlighted the prejudice towards homeopathy among resident doctors attending the University of Campinas Medical School. Eighty-six (49%) out of 176 rejected homeopathy as a discipline in the medical curriculum, affirming that there is not enough scientific evidence to support this practice.

Acupuncture was recognised as a medical specialty in 1995, and in 2002 the Ministry of Education created a Medical Residency Programme in acupuncture. Currently, the programme consists of 5,760 hours with a duration of two years, and runs in nine higher education institutions across the country (*Colégio Médico Brasileiro de Acupuntura*, 2012). In 2012, acupuncture was regulated by the National Agency of Supplementary Health – a regulatory agency from the Ministry of Health responsible for regulating health insurance plan operators, service providers and users – as a 'multiprofessional practice', extending the regulation of this therapy's use to physiotherapists, occupational therapists, phonoaudiologists, dental surgeons, nurses, pharmacists, psychologists and nutritionists (*Conselho Nacional de Saúde*, 2012). Finally, as previously mentioned, in 2006, anthroposophical medicine was approved as a medical observatory within the SUS, with the aim of guiding national policy. Most medical doctors practising anthroposophical medicine have acquired postgraduate training, which only exists in one private institution – that of the Brazilian Association of Anthroposophic Medicine (*Associação Brasileira de Medicina Antroposófica*).

Clearly, medical doctors and allied health care professionals have been trying to co-opt and incorporate CAM, monopolising CAM within the SUS and thus excluding traditional CAM practitioners from practice within the public sector. Yet the incorporation of specific CAM therapies into the Brazilian medical canon has created problems for allied health care professionals as well, who are authorised by their professional bodies to practise CAM, but are discredited by the medical associations (Nascimento et al, 2013). Furthermore, as previously indicated, the regulation of these practices as medical specialties has created problems within the medical profession itself, which is divided between those who have practised CAM within the SUS, and those who disbelieve in its practice.

It is thus not surprising that the 2006 Brazilian policy on CAM caused uproar among most medical doctors (*Conselho Federal de Medicina*, 2006). The concern of the Brazilian Federal Medical Council (CFM) about the plethora of professionals working in the health care field, without a clear definition of the limits to their professional practice, has increased over the years. The Medical Act 2013, expressed in Bills 268/2002 and 7703/2006, was a reflection of that concern. It aimed at regulating medical activities and exerting pressure for social closure, granting privileges to the medical profession. After long discussions in the upper and lower houses of Congress, both Bills were compiled into Act 12.842/2013, and approved by ex-President Dilma Rousseff, who vetoed some paragraphs, on 10 July 2013. The reasons for such vetoes were various, including that Act 12.842/2013 promoted a caring model that is strongly medically centred, and was based on strong medical corporate power; and that there was an overestimation of hierarchical medical services, with greater importance of certain activities over others. Ex-President Rousseff's vetoes were thus justified through the multiprofessional principle of the SUS (Cabral, 2013). The Medical Act and this study thereby exemplify the existing wedge between CAM and the medical profession.

Nevertheless, the number of CAM practitioners (biomedically and non-biomedically qualified) and CAM consultations has increased in both the public and private sectors. In the public health service, the Health Ministry's newsletter from November 2016 reports that almost two million visits to a CAM practitioner in 1,582 municipalities, in more than 3,248 primary health care centres, were registered from January to August of 2016 (Ministry of Health of Brazil, 2016). Furthermore, in September 2016, 5,848 health care services had offered complementary and alternative practices (PIC), and 202 were primary health care centres and 203 were hospitals, thus showing the transversality of the policy. The most popular practices have been traditional Chinese medicine, followed by other practices not contemplated by the 2006 Act (Ministry of Health of Brazil, 2016). This last aspect raises the question of whether the state governance of CAM within the SUS has been in accord with the interests of the public, since the latter have turned to CAM practices other than those included in the 2006 policy document.

It is interesting to observe that those professionals who use CAM and work in the public sector have extended control over their practice but limited governance; while those who work in the private sector have almost no control over their practice although they have full governance through voluntary professional associations with regulatory powers granted by the state. The number of these associations offering professional safety and quality standards and legal advice to begin and protect the practice of a variety of CAM therapies has increased since the end of the 1990s. Examples are the Trade Union of Natural Therapists (SINATEN) and the Holistic Therapists Council of Brazil (OTHB), both founded in 1996, the National Association of Therapists (ANT) created in 2003, the National Federation of Therapists (FENATE) founded in 2004, and the Brazilian Association of Holistic Therapists (ABRATH) created in 2007, all with the aim of regulating the 'holistic therapist' professional in Brazil. According to the International Society of Therapists (*Sociedade Internacional de Terapistas*, 2016), there are around 150,000 professionals working in holistic therapy, including acupuncturists, floral therapists, herbal therapists, aestheticians, body therapists, chiropractors, orthomolecular therapists and reiki therapists.

To conclude, CAM practice in Brazil has increased since the creation of the SUS, both within the SUS and the private sector. A set of regulatory Acts governing CAM practice within the SUS has been created, although almost no statutory regulation for CAM practice outside the SUS exists. Furthermore, the underfunding of SUS, after 28 years of existence, is still a big concern. In 2016, since the governmental shift towards right-wing ideologies after the impeachment of ex-President Rousseff, the Ministry of Health has intended to reduce the health budget (Bezerra, 2016). As economic and political issues are intertwined, the biggest challenge for the survival of the SUS and CAM policies is thus political. The next section looks at recent modes of CAM governance in Portugal.

CAM governance in Portugal

Portugal has been a constitutional democratic republic since the Carnation revolution (*Revolução dos Cravos*) in 1974, which ended 41 years of dictatorship in the country. Portugal was the first European colonial power as well as the last Western European country to release its colonies (Fischer and Klatte, 2011). In 1975, the country accepted the independence of most of its former colonies, although Brazil had already become independent in 1822.

The Portuguese National Health System (*Sistema Nacional de Saúde*, SNS) was established in 1979, after the revolution and a period of restructuring of health care services. The SNS provides universal health care coverage, is mainly tax-financed and so has a mix of public and private funding (Barros et al, 2011). Health care delivery is based on both public and private providers and approximately 20% to 25% of the population enjoy extra layers of health insurance coverage through health subsystems (specific insurance schemes for certain professions, such as the ADSE, a social health insurance system for public sector employees and their dependents), and 10% to 20% of the population have voluntary health insurance. The Portuguese Ministry of Health (*Ministério da Saúde*) and its agencies are in charge of managing the SNS.

CAM governance in Portugal has had a peculiar narrative. To begin with, the recommended term 'traditional and complementary medicine' of the WHO (2000) is not used in CAM affairs in the country; the term 'non-conventional therapeutics' is the one mainly used. In the same way as in Brazil, this 'linguistic twist' has been the result of a long political and professional battle between the state, the medical profession and CAM practitioners.

State interest in CAM began in the late 1990s, when a report on the legal status of CAM produced by a working group made up of representatives appointed by the Ministry of Health was published (*Direção Geral de Saúde*, 1999). This report advised that CAM should be regulated in the country, and highlighted the spread of a diversity of perspectives within health care worldwide. This document, however, was a source of discord between the state, the medical profession (along with other allied health care professions) and CAM practitioners, and marked the beginning of a bargaining process between these three actors concerning CAM regulation (Almeida and Gabe, 2016).

After an enduring dispute among different political parties, which helped to reinforce the fragmentary nature of the state, Act 45/2003 was passed. This Act statutorily regulated six CAM therapies – acupuncture, homeopathy, osteopathy, chiropractic, naturopathy and phytotherapy – and put them on the road to professionalisation (*Assembleia da República Portuguesa*, 2003). An ad-hoc committee was subsequently created and charged with legislating on the competencies and credentialism of each of these therapies. This committee, however, never finished its work, as many representatives of biomedical disciplines resigned (Almeida and Gabe, 2016). Furthermore, CAM practitioners engaged in peer battles themselves as regards CAM regulation, thus exposing to the public, the media and other professions a significant lack of cohesion and collegiality (Almeida, 2012). It took 10 years for the state to intervene in this process, after much pressure from left-wing political parties such as the Left Block, which submitted letters to the government, recommending the completion of CAM regulation in the country. The governmental response to such pressures resulted in the new Act 71/2013, which replaced Act 45/2003 and added one more therapy, traditional Chinese medicine, to the list of CAM therapies to be regulated – an action much contested by the Medical Council at the time.

Since Act 71/2013, CAM regulation has developed. A second ad-hoc committee was set up and in October 2014 the government published the competencies for the seven CAM therapies included in Act 71/2013. More recently, in June 2015, the government published the educational standards of five out of the seven therapies included in the new Act. These documents recognise acupuncture, osteopathy, chiropractic, phytotherapy and naturopathy, thus excluding homeopathy and traditional Chinese medicine, and set the educational standards for becoming a CAM professional, which involve completion of a four-year higher education degree within the polytechnic system (Almeida and Gabe, 2016). In October 2015, 17 CAM BSc programme proposals were submitted to the A3ES, the Portuguese state agency for the assessment and accreditation of higher education institutions and their study programmes, yet only five – all on osteopathy – have been approved (Leiria, 2016). Osteopathy has therefore been at the forefront of 'academic' CAM in the country, having launched its BSc programmes in September 2016 within the polytechnic system.

The changes in CAM regulation in Portugal over the past decades, however, have been accompanied by shifts in the responses of the Medical Council towards CAM practice. First, in the late 1990s, when the state manifested interest in governing CAM, the Medical Council's response towards CAM therapies was one of rejection. For example, the council's representatives of the working group and the first ad-hoc committee to legislate on CAM resigned, due to disagreements on policy making and incompatibilities with other members of the group, particularly with CAM representatives (Almeida and Gabe, 2016). Second, the Medical Council vehemently and successfully opposed the use of the word 'medicine' by CAM practitioners, proposing in one of its reports (*Secção Regional do Norte da Ordem dos Médicos*, 2001) the replacement of the term 'complementary and alternative medicine' with the term 'non-conventional therapeutics'. Yet the Medical Council did not have the same success in its claim to replace the term 'traditional Chinese medicine' with 'traditional Chinese therapies', and the former has prevailed in policy documents.

A main argument by the Portuguese Medical Council about CAM regulation has been the lack of scientific evidence for these therapies, homeopathy being the most controversial in this respect (*Secção Regional do Norte da Ordem dos Médicos*, 2001). By the end of the 1990s, CAM therapies and practitioners had been associated with 'charlatanism' and 'quackery' by the Medical Council (Bessa, 1999). Yet in 2002 the council granted medical status to acupuncture. Acupuncture started being incorporated into the postgraduate medical curriculum and in 2002 the Portuguese Society of Medical Acupuncture was founded. In the same way as acupuncture in Brazil, there was an attempt to incorporate acupuncture into Portuguese medicine, by converting it into a biomedical therapeutic and separating it from its traditional roots.

There is a lack of data on the use of CAM by the lay populace in Portugal, and the grassroots movements in CAM have been weak. According to the International Social Survey Programme Research Group (2015), 81.7% of the Portuguese population have never visited an alternative health care practitioner. Nevertheless, recent research has suggested that more than two million people regularly seek CAM in the country (*Federação Nacional de Associações de Medicinas Alternativas Naturais*, 2008). Furthermore, Tavares (2015) has shown that people tend to use CAM concomitantly with conventional Western medicine, both in the diagnosis and treatment stages. The more empowered the patients are too, the more likely they are to choose CAM; therefore, suffering from chronic conditions and holding higher levels of education tend to be determinant factors in choosing CAM treatments in Portugal.

It is clear that the legal status of CAM in Portugal has changed in recent years, largely due to the manifest interest of the state in governing such therapies, for which CAM associations and leaders actively lobbied during the late 1990s. The seven specific CAM professions have shifted from voluntary self-regulation and occupational professionalism, where discretion and control existed within each occupational group, to state exclusionary closure and increasing organisational professionalism, where there are rational-legal and bureaucratic forms of authority, including by the state, that have controlled their work (Evetts, 2013). This shift makes Portugal a pioneer European country in having such an extensive statutory legislation framework for CAM. Furthermore, the position of Portugal within Europe and the wider world in relation to CAM legislation can potentially facilitate cross-border health care opportunities in the CAM field, and turn Portugal itself into a CAM treatment, training and practice country.

Statutory regulation, however, may have unintended consequences for CAM therapies themselves, and for the wider public. The discourse of professionalism coming from the state has appealed to CAM practitioners in Portugal since the 1990s, and it has been perceived as a way of improving their status, power and financial rewards in the country (Almeida, 2016). However, the extent to which acquiring statutory regulation has benefited, or will benefit, CAM professionals and/or the broader public has been an issue of concern among the CAM community since Act 71/2013. In other words, is statutory regulation of CAM necessarily aligned with CAM professionals and the public interest in Portugal?

First, state regulation has provided protection to CAM practitioners from threats from the public and other health care professions, but has also implied less occupational control, autonomy and participation in the make-up of their profession. The Portuguese government, through its agencies, decides how and which CAM professionals should be regulated, their professional conduct, and the extent and modes of use of CAM. The government can also withdraw the authorisation given to CAM professionals if the law is violated. Furthermore, Act 71/2013 clearly lays down the content of BSc programmes in CAM and the 2015 state directives for the educational standards of five CAM therapies give clear indications of the discipline areas that these therapies should incorporate in their curriculum. Thus, professionalism from above can be seen as a powerful ideology, the effects of which are not the occupational control and autonomy of CAM professionals over their work, but rather disciplinary control, or control 'at a distance', by the state and its institutions – thus limiting the exercise by CAM practitioners of discretionary decision making (Evetts, 2013).

Second, professionalism from above also brings the standardisation of knowledge and practice, which on the one hand can bring a sense of common expertise and occupational identity among all statutorily regulated CAM professions. However, on the other, it can threaten the highly diverse field of CAM and its philosophy. For example, Act 71/2013 and subsequent directives for CAM's educational standards stipulate training in 'fundamental sciences' (such as anatomy and biology) and 'clinical techniques and science' (such as pathology, epidemiology and public health) across the five CAM therapies – acupuncture, osteopathy, chiropractic, phytotherapy and naturopathy (*Assembleia da República Portuguesa*, 2013). There has thus been an attempt to standardise education across all five regulated therapies, which can lead to disenchantment, not only among potential CAM recruits, but also among the wider public. Yet the standardisation and harmonisation of knowledge and practice associated with professionalism from above may supply predictability to the public and consequently improve the relationship of trust between CAM practitioners and their clients/patients (Evetts, 2011).

Finally, being statutorily regulated has not necessarily meant employment in the public sector or the democratisation of access to these therapies. Although CAM regulation in the country has put seven CAM therapies on the road to professionalisation, CAM practice has mainly remained outside the SNS and CAM services and is mainly provided in the private, free market, paid directly and fully by the patient in a fee-for-service system or co-paid by private health care insurance schemes such as Multicare and Medicare, which tend to only cover CAM treatments prescribed by medical doctors with additional training and education in CAM (Tavares, 2015).

Conclusion

Clearly, the status of CAM and CAM practitioners has changed in Brazil and Portugal since the 1980s. Brazil and Portugal, as two countries with a longstanding economic, political and cultural relationship, have presented various similarities. Both implemented free public health care services – the SUS and the SNS – established during the second half of the 20th century, after the dismantlement of dictatorships. Subsequently, both countries have followed WHO recommendations and guidelines for the creation of national policies to govern CAM: Brazil created Act 971 in 2006, which regulates homeopathy, traditional Chinese medicine/acupuncture, phytotherapy, social thermalism/chrenotherapy and anthroposophical medicine within the SUS; Portugal created Act 71/2013, which replaced Act 45/2003, and regulates the professional activity of homeopathy, acupuncture, traditional Chinese medicine, phytotherapy, osteopathy, chiropractic and naturopathy. Both countries have therefore taken into account the social values of justice, general welfare and freedom in the governance of their health care, and to this extent they have functioned in the public interest.

In Brazil, specific CAM therapies have been statutorily regulated to be practised by medical doctors and other allied health care professionals within the SUS. Yet CAM practitioners outside the SUS have remained statutorily unregulated and therefore governed by their own professional bodies. In Portugal, in turn, the CAM presence and use by medical doctors and allied health care professionals in the SNS is less marked, as the state has focused more on regulating CAM professionals than therapies. Yet CAM therapies have also been regulated and incorporated into the medical curriculum. In fact, both countries have seen the co-optation (Baer and Coulter, 2008) or incorporation (Saks, 1995) of some CAM therapies – acupuncture, homeopathy and anthroposophical medicine became medical specialties and 'multiprofessional' practices in Brazil, while 'medical acupuncture' is offered at postgraduate medical level in Portugal. Both countries have also changed the name of their national policies throughout the regulation process, banning the word 'medicine' present in previous versions of state documents. The provision of CAM by medical doctors and allied health care professionals has therefore conflicted with CAM practitioners' interests, as it tends to diminish the need for their professionalisation and existence.

In Brazil, CAM practitioners, who hold professional self-regulatory status, have had the freedom to control their practice and work conditions through their professional bodies. Yet they have no protection from the state and, although they have successfully manipulated the private CAM market, they have had to compete with health care professionals within the SUS who have acquired training in CAM that is sponsored by the state and use CAM therapies in their professional practice. This segregation of CAM practitioners into the private CAM market has put them in a vulnerable position, preventing them from acquiring higher status, power, influence and authority within health care. The role of various voluntary self-regulatory bodies in fighting for legislation for CAM practitioners and claiming to serve the public interest in terms of practitioner credentials and service quality is thus distinct in Brazil. Yet, as Adams (2016) states, professional self-regulation has been in decline worldwide due to changing meanings of the public interest, despite being an economic bargain for governments, as professionals support their professional bodies through registration fees.

In Portugal, on the contrary, state regulation has appealed to CAM practitioners as a mechanism to promote and facilitate CAM's occupational closure since the late 1990s. With Act 71/2013, Portugal shifted to a social closure regulated system, and a state discourse rich in objectives and ideologies has acted as a disciplinary mechanism over CAM. The state has regulated seven CAM professions, even if these are not generally included in the delivery of the public health care system. Although CAM practitioners have undoubtedly achieved professional recognition and protection of their titles, there has been a fear within the CAM community of losing occupational control of their work over time, and consequently of losing their shared identity and limiting professional discretion and expert judgement in the name of bureaucracy and standardisation.

Furthermore, the rhetoric of science has been used by the state to set standards of practice within the SUS and standards of education within the higher education system in Portugal. As Evetts (2013: 790) has put it, 'in effect, professionalism is being used to convince, cajole and persuade employees, practitioners and other workers to perform and behave in ways which the organisation or institution [the state] deems to be appropriate, effective and efficient'. Consequently, in the case of Portugal, the shift from collegiate to bureaucratic ways of organising CAM practitioners' work might lead to neglecting CAM clients' interests, since organisational professionalism usually leads to a deterioration of professional values and so to 'malpractice' (Evetts, 2011), and also to a disenchantment of practitioner–client relations and a disempowerment of the practitioner over the client.

In sum, Brazil and Portugal illustrate two cases of countries that have created national policies on CAM and therefore attempted to maintain the principles of universality, integrality and equality established by their own constitutions and by supra-state agencies such as the WHO. However, although both countries have met some aspects of the WHO (2013) traditional medicine strategy for 2014-23, CAM policy is a process still in progress, facing challenges and uncertainties particularly in relation to serving and protecting the interests of the public and CAM practitioners; in respect of the latter, the main challenge is either to the interests of those who hold more informal educational credentials, like many CAM practitioners in Brazil, or to those who have had educational standards and practice guidelines imposed by the state, such as the case of CAM practitioners in Portugal.

References

Adams, T. L. (2016) 'Professional self-regulation and the public interest in Canada', *Professions and Professionalism* 6(2), https://journals.hioa. no/index.php/pp/article/view/1587/1586

Almeida, J. (2012) 'The differential incorporation of CAM into the medical establishment: the case of acupuncture and homeopathy in Portugal', *Health Sociology Review* 21(1): 5-22.

Almeida, J. (2016) 'Complementary and alternative medicine's occupational closure in Portuguese healthcare: contradictions and challenges', *Health: An Interdisciplinary Journal for the Social Study of Health, Illness and Medicine* 20(5): 447-64.

Almeida, J and Gabe, J. (2016) 'CAM within a field force of countervailing powers: the case of Portugal', *Social Science and Medicine* 155: 73-81.

Assembleia da República Portuguesa (2003) 'Lei no 45/2003 de 22 de Agosto: lei do enquadramento base das terapêuticas não convencionais: I serie A', *Diário da Assembleia da República* 193: 5391-2.

Assembleia da República Portuguesa (2013) 'Lei no 71/2013 de 2 de Setembro: Regulamenta a lei 45/2003, de 22 de Agosto, relativamente ao exercício profissional das atividades de aplicação de terapêuticas não convencionais: I serie', *Diário da Assembleia da República* 168: 5439-42.

Baer, H. A. and Coulter, I. D. (2008) 'Taking stock of integrative medicine: broadening biomedicine or co-option of complementary and alternative medicine?', *Health Sociology Review* 17(4): 331-41.

Bahia, L. (2009) 'Sistema Único de Saúde', *Dicionário da Educação Profissional em Saúde*, Fundação Oswaldo Cruz, Escola Politécnica de Saúde Joaquim Venâncio, www.epsjv.fiocruz.br/dicionario/verbetes/sisunisau.html

Barros, P. P., Machado, S. R. and Simões, J. A. (2011) 'Portugal health system review', in World Health Organization, *European Observatory on Health Systems and Policies*, Denmark: WHO Regional Office for Europe.

Bessa, P. (1999) 'A ordem dos médicos não vai participar na regulamentação de falsas medicinas', *Primeiro de Janeiro* 27 July: 5.

Bezerra, A. (2016) '"O maior desafio do SUS é politico", afirma Jairnilson Paim, em aula aberta na Fiocruz', Rio de Janeiro: ICICT/Fiocruz, 3 May, www.icict.fiocruz.br/content/%E2%80%9Co-maior-desafio-do-sus-%C3%A9-pol%C3%ADtico%E2%80%9D-afirma-jairnilson-paim-em-aula-aberta-na-fiocruz

Brosnan, C. (2015) '"Quackery" in the academy? Professional knowledge, autonomy and the debate over complementary medicine degrees', *Sociology* 49(6): 1047-64.

Brosnan, C. (2016) 'Epistemic cultures in complementary medicine: knowledge-making in university departments of osteopathy and Chinese medicine', *Health Sociology Review* 25(2): 171-86.

Burns, E. B. (1993) *A History of Brazil*, New York, NY: Columbia University Press.

Cabral, I. E. (2013) 'Statement of the Brazilian nursing association regarding the approval of the medical practice act', *Revista Brasileira de Enfermagem* 66(4): 469-70.

Cant, S. and Sharma, U. (1999) *A New Medical Pluralism? Alternative Medicine, Doctors, Patients and the State*, London: UCL Press.

Chamber of Deputies Directing Board (2010) *Constitution of the Federative Republic of Brazil*, Brazil: Documentation and Information Centre.

Colégio Médico Brasileiro de Acupuntura (2012) 'No Brasil, a residência médica em acupuntura tem carga horária de 5.760 horas, durante dois anos, em nove universidades do país', *Colégio Médico de Acupuntura Webpage*, 25 July, www.maxpressnet.com. br/Conteudo/1,516155,No_Brasil_a_residencia_medica_em_ Acupuntura_tem_carga_horaria_de_5760_horas_durante_dois_anos_ em_nove_universidades_do_p,516155,9.htm

Conrad, P. (2007) *The Medicalization of Society: On the Transformation of Human Conditions into Treatable Disorders*, Baltimore, MD: Johns Hopkins University Press.

Conselho Federal de Medicina (2006) 'Saúde não é moeda de negociação política', *Conselho Federal de Medicina Webpage*, http://portal.cfm.org. br/index.php?option=com_content&view=article&id=20276&cati d=46:artigos&Itemid=18

Conselho Nacional de Saúde (2012) *Resolução n° 463/12*, 12 December.

de Barros, N. F. and Fiuza, A. R. (2014) 'Medicina baseada em evidência e medicina baseada em preconceito: o caso da homeopatia', *Cadernos de Saúde Pública* 30(11): 2368-76.

Direção Geral de Saúde (1999) 'Medicinas não convencionais', *Relatório do Grupo de Trabalho*, Lisbon, 16 March.

Evetts, J. (2011) 'A new professionalism? Challenges and opportunities', *Current Sociology* 59(4): 406-22.

Evetts, J. (2013) 'Professionalism: value and ideology', *Current Sociology* 61(5/6): 778-96.

Federação Nacional de Associações de Medicinas Alternativas Naturais (2008) 'Editorial', *Boletim da Federação*, February, 1(2).

Fischer, M. and Klatte, S. (2011) 'Decolonisation: Portuguese territories', *Max Planck Encyclopaedia of Public International Law*, Oxford: Oxford University Press.

Givati, A. (2015) 'Performing "pragmatic holism": professionalisation and the holistic discourse of non-medically qualified acupuncturists and homeopaths in the United Kingdom', *Health: An Interdisciplinary Journal for the Social Study of Health, Illness and Medicine* 19(1): 34-50.

Givati A. and Hatton, K. (2015) 'Traditional acupuncturists and higher education in Britain: the dual, paradoxical impact of biomedical alignment on the holistic view', *Social Science and Medicine* 131: 173-80.

Ijaz, N., Boon, H., Muzzin, L. and Welsh, S. (2016) 'State risk discourse and the regulatory preservation of traditional medicine knowledge: the case of acupuncture in Ontario, Canada', *Social Science and Medicine* 170: 97-105.

International Social Survey Programme Research Group (2015) *International Social Survey Programme: Health and Healthcare – ISSP 2011*, Cologne: GESIS Data Archive.

Leiria, I. (2016) 'Medicinas alternativas não chegam ao superior', *Expresso*, Secção Sociedade, 28 May.

Ministry of Health of Brazil (1999) Portaria no 1.230, *Diário Oficial da União*, 14 October, no 199-E, Seção 1: 12-158, http://bvsms.saude.gov.br/bvs/saudelegis/gm/1999/anexo/anexoprt1230_14_10_1999.pdf

Ministry of Health of Brazil (2006) Portaria n° 971/06: Aprova a Política Nacional de Práticas Integrativas e Complementares (PNPIC) no Sistema Único de Saúde, *Diário Oficial da União*, 3 May, Seção 1: 20-25, www.crbm1.gov.br/Portaria%20MS%20971%202006.pdf

Ministry of Health of Brazil (2008) *National Policy on Integrative and Complementary Practices of the SUS*, Brazil: Ministry of Health of Brazil, http://189.28.128.100/dab/docs/publicacoes/geral/pnpic_ingles.pdf

Ministry of Health of Brazil (2016) 'Informe Novembro', *Newsletter*, Ministry of Health of Brazil, http://189.28.128.100/dab/docs/portaldab/documentos/informe_novembro_PICS.pdf

Monteiro, D. A. and Iriart, J. A. B. (2007) 'Homeopatia no sistema único de saúde: representações dos usuários sobre o tratamento homeopático', *Cadernos de Saúde Pública* 23(8): 1903-12.

Nascimento, M. C., Barros, N. F., Nogueira, M. I. and Luz, M. T. (2013) 'A categoria racionalidade médica e uma nova epistemologia em saúde', *Ciência & Saúde Coletiva* 18(12): 3595-604.

Paim, J., Travassos, C., Almeida, C., Bahia, L. and Macinko, J. (2011) 'The Brazilian health system: history, advances, and challenges', *The Lancet* 377: 1778-97.

Parkin, F. (1979) *Marxism and Class Theory: A Bourgeois Critique*, London: Tavistock Publications.

Saks, M. (1995) *Professions and the Public Interest: Medical Power, Altruism and Alternative Medicine*, London: Routledge.

Saks, M. (2012) 'Defining a profession: the role of knowledge and expertise', *Professions and Professionalism* 2: 1-10.

Saks, M. (2015a) 'Health policy and complementary and alternative medicine', in Kuhlmann, E., Blank, R. H., Bourgeault, I. L. and Wendt, C. (eds) *The Palgrave International Handbook of Healthcare Policy and Governance*, Basingstoke: Palgrave Macmillan: 494-509.

Saks, M. (2015b) *The Professions, State and the Market: Medicine in Britain, the United States and Russia*, London: Routledge.

Secção Regional do Norte da Ordem dos Médicos (2001) 'Actividades desenvolvidas pela SRNOM: Parecer da Ordem dos Médicos sobre os projetos de diplomas reguladores do exercício das medicinas não convencionais apresentado à Comissão Parlamentar de Saúde', *NorteMédico – Revista da Secção Regional do Norte Ordem dos Médicos* 8(3): 50-1.

Sociedade Internacional de Terapistas (2016) *Conceitos Gerais*, www.sinte. com.br/faq/index.php?action=artikel&cat=14&id=96&artlang= pt-br

Tavares, A. I. (2015) 'Substitutes or complements? Diagnosis and treatment with non-conventional and conventional medicine', *International Journal of Health Policy and Management* 4(4): 235-42.

WHO (World Health Organization) (1978) 'Declaration of Alma-Ata', International Conference on Primary Health Care, Alma-Ata, USSR, 6-12 September.

WHO (2000) *General Guidelines for Methodologies on Research and Evaluation of Traditional Medicine*, Geneva: WHO.

WHO (2002) *World Health Organization's Traditional Medicine Strategy 2002-2005*, Geneva: WHO.

WHO (2013) *WHO Traditional Medicine Strategy: 2014-2023*, Geneva: WHO.

ELEVEN

Birth of the hydra-headed monster: a unique antipodean model of health workforce governance

Fiona Pacey and Stephanie Short

Introduction

Just as an individual may occupy many roles in relation to health care (patient, consumer, carer, health practitioner, taxpayer and citizen), likewise the organisation that is responsible for health practitioner regulation needs to be responsive to a series of different audiences. In terms of individuals, this includes patients for whom a safe outcome is sought and practitioners who are the subject of the regulatory oversight. Taking a wider view, the community expects the organisation to act in the interests of patients over the professions, and indeed other parties including governments. The governments that establish the legislative framework and regulatory agencies expect that the organisation will effectively undertake the tasks assigned to it, as just outlined, in such a manner that promotes confidence in the provision of health care – irrespective of how it is delivered or funded.

However, what happens when the same governments that are responsible for establishing a regulatory agency also become collectively accountable for that organisation when they only have the authority to act individually? How can governance arrangements be conceptualised in such circumstances? And what effect does this have on the relationships between the state, health professions and the public that they are responsible to? This chapter seeks to answer this set of questions in the context of the development of historic health workforce regulatory reform in Australia. In Australia the National Scheme for the Registration and Accreditation of the Health Professions led to the establishment of a new structure and creation – in effect a clean state – that drew on existing local thinking and expertise (Carlton, 2005; Healy and Braithwaite, 2006), as well as reforms pursued elsewhere (Rogers, 2004; Pacey et al, 2017). In

2016, the national scheme oversaw the regulation of 14 professional groups and in excess of 650,000 registered individuals, equating to almost 3% of the Australian population (Australian Health Practitioner Regulation Agency, 2016). In the intergovernmental agreement that blueprinted the national scheme in July 2010, a series of objectives was anchored around the protection of the public and wider health workforce governance concerns.

This chapter focuses on analysing the context in which these objectives were designed, within the wider context of the society, the state and professions. It does not seek to assess the efficacy of the regulatory instruments that the national scheme implemented, nor the actions they undertake to achieve those objectives. Specifically, we examine how the governance and oversight arrangements of the scheme provide an accountability framework that is both responsive and responsible to the community, through its elected governments. And, as we will explore in more detail, that accountability responds to risks evident in a wider political and social frame.

Australia is an island continent with a population of 24 million people who predominately live in urban centres within one hour of the coastline. It has a federal system of government, a written constitution and, apart from its first peoples (Aboriginal and Torres Strait Islanders), a life expectancy of its population of over 80 years. The majority of health professionals are educated in publicly funded universities, and work in public, not-for-profit and private settings, including as independent practitioners. Both the federal and state and territory governments are involved in the funding and provision of health care services. Approximately 70% of all funds spent on health care in Australia are held by government. At the national level, funds are sourced from consolidated funds, as well as a levy applied to individuals – 'the Medicare levy' (Palmer and Short, 2014). As the six state and two territory governments have less income-raising capacity and hold responsibility for the delivery of services across key areas of health, education and transport, they also receive allocations from the federal government.

In Australia's dry and sparsely populated continent, the distribution of the health workforce across regional, rural and remote areas remains problematic, and a range of interventions has been developed including around health professionals in training to address maldistribution challenges (Mason, 2013). However, these underserved areas continue to be reliant on overseas trained doctors, nurses and allied health practitioners (Negin et al, 2013). It was from the context of health services and regulatory bodies responding to shortages and associated pressures that emerged one of the most infamous instances of regulatory failure in Australia, the Patel scandal at Bundaberg Hospital, which saw a series of significant adverse clinical outcomes following the registration (and internal promotion) of a practitioner who had not disclosed restrictions on a medical licence in the United States (US) (Pacey et al, 2010).

The National Scheme for the Registration and Accreditation of the Health Professions in Australia (the scheme) was a policy initiative (enacted by legislative means) designed to improve regulatory arrangements, especially through consistency across all state and territory jurisdictions in a federal system of government (see Table 11.1). It initially covered 10 professions (chiropractors, dental practitioners, medical practitioners, nurses and midwives, optometrists, osteopaths, pharmacists, physiotherapists, podiatrists and psychologists) when it commenced in 2010. Four further professions (Aboriginal and Torres Strait Islander health practitioners, Chinese medicine practitioners, medical radiation practitioners and occupational therapists) were added to the scheme in 2014.

Table 11.1: The Australian jurisdictions

		Population (as at 30 June 2015)
Northern Territory	Territory	0.24 million
Australian Capital Territory	Territory	0.39 million
Tasmania	State	0.52 million
South Australia	State	1.7 million
Western Australia	State	2.6 million
Queensland	State	4.8 million
Victoria	State	5.9 million
New South Wales	State	7.6 million
Australia	Commonwealth	23.8 million

Source: Population figures are drawn from the Australian Bureau of Statistics, catalogue number 3235.0, Population by Age and Sex, Regions of Australia, www.abs.gov.au/ausstats/abs@.nsf/mf/3235.0

A national challenge

Prior to the birth of the scheme, there was different legislation in each state and territory and around 80 different agencies were responsible for the registration of individual health practitioners and of the accreditation of the education that leads to registration. In practical terms, there was inconsistency in which professions were regulated in different states and territories and in the requirements in each, including the level of information included on public registers (that is, whether or not specialty qualifications were listed in the case of medical and some other practitioners). The separate requirements were especially an issue for practitioners who lived in communities that straddled across different states or territories and were therefore required to maintain two sets of registration. There were also significant inconsistences in the second aspect of the scheme – the accreditation of education and training required in each profession to meet the registration standards. These ranged from strongly developed and performed by profession affiliated organisations, to those that had no existing processes. The design enabled the former to be delegated to undertake those activities under the scheme, while others had to establish new authorities (Australian Health Ministers' Advisory Council, 2014).

This chapter examines these recent regulatory changes in Australia and how the changes were designed to enable multiple governments to continue to be involved in the management of health workforce regulation, as expected by the community or public (which in a democracy is represented but not restricted to the voting public). First, we articulate the context of the public interest as used throughout this chapter. It is not one that is focusing on the professions acting in the public interest (Saks, 2015), but rather is concerned with the actions undertaken by governments, initially as designers of a new regulatory regime and subsequently as core to its governance. This reflects an explicit desire for governments to maintain their influence in health workforce governance, with an explicit recognition that the regulation is of a market – and one which, while delivering services to individuals, also has wider societal implications. In Australia, this has been described by Haines (2011: 86), a criminologist, as a manifestation of an improvement regime: 'The "invisible hand" of the market ... disciplined by the visible, accountable and transparent hand of the regulator.' As Haines goes on further to observe, in such a design endeavour governments are conscious of managing their political risk through providing reassurance that regulation delivers the safety sought by the community, while not excessively restricting economic growth, recognising that both factors are part of the expectations of governments by their communities. And from Haines, whose work is examining the context of regulation, we will also move through some of the literature relating to the roles of government in health workforce planning and management, and specifically where they undertake regulatory activities as one of those roles.

Increasingly, governments are engaging in rhetoric about protecting the security of citizens in a complex global environment and safety is the element that policy, legislative and other actions are designed to assure. But safety (to one's life and physical wellbeing) is not only compromised by the fear and actuality of terrorist or other violent acts, it can also be caused by more universal and familiar experiences. In the experience of health care, with its complications of individual and system error, there are substantial safety concerns (Kohn et al, 2000). The implications of errors are not just a concern for patients or their families – the community as a whole shoulders costs, whether through increased fees of practitioners generated by insurance premiums or through loss of taxation by individuals and potentially costs of further treatment or additional care, as well as non-economic costs.

The World Health Organization (2017) describes the manner in which governments undertake activities to support the wellbeing of their populations (including regulation) as governance (or stewardship). The notion of governance is one that is supportive of governments acting in a current and future context and the need to consider cautious endeavours, as well as ones of innovation, in designing and delivering environments and institutions – whether through regulatory or operational measures. This notion sits well alongside the introduction of the National Scheme for the Registration and Accreditation of the Health Professions, which was designed in the context of recognising finite resources, in the case of both funding and workforce, and a need to improve the consistency of the experience for all Australians, irrespective of the state or territory in which they live.

We now outline the changes that were introduced under the scheme, and briefly examine the reasons for its introduction and the existing challenges that governments and the community have been facing, which the scheme was intended to address. Second, we explain the complex legislative and governance arrangements that were required to operationalise the scheme, and explore the level of complexity that was required to ensure that governments could maintain their involvement in health workforce regulation. Finally, we consider the accountability framework that these arrangements established and investigate whether these act in the public interest. And, we will also adopt the use of a metaphor as championed by Liljegren and Saks (2016) and others, and represent the nine Australian governments – and more specifically their health ministers – as a hydra-headed monster, an ancient mythical creature that serves as a proxy for a formidable foe being represented physically by many (often nine) heads. This representation will be creatively, yet deliberatively contemplated in considering especially the distributed and diffused nature of government responsibility and accountability for the new national regulatory scheme.

Professions, governments and managerialism

There has been significant exploration about the changing relationships between the professions and the state in the recent decades globally. It is recognised that much of this literature relates predominately, but not exclusively, to medical practitioners. This reflects existing professional hierarchies as evident in Australia and elsewhere, reflected in both financial reward and level of autonomy and influence on the health and broader policy environment. For our purposes, the literature is considered thematically and is not used universally – and is not aiming to differentiate between professions. Indeed, this is consistent with one of the notable features of the national scheme in Australia, which has seen the inclusion of medical practitioners, on the same basis as all other professions, under the scheme. This outcome was not without some disagreement, particularly among some medical stakeholders, but pointed to drivers of regulatory change that were not exclusively directed towards one professional group.

There has been transnational examination of the changing relationship between the state and the professions in the regulatory space, with an increasing inclusion of patients as consumers of health services becoming a stronger presence, whether as a reflexive conceptual response or a tangible presence in regulatory arrangements (Salter, 2003; Kuhlmann and Saks, 2008; Healy, 2011; Kuhlmann and Larsen, 2015). Other sociologists have acknowledged the context of the professions as part of the apparatus of the state, including as interpreters and guides at a time when scientific knowledge and medical information have become both more accessible and more complex within a risk society paradigm (Chamberlain, 2013).

The influence of managerialism, particularly relating to those health practitioners undertaking clinical practice in an institutional setting, has also been canvassed. Some of these studies have been investigating responses by professions to increased oversight through reporting (Waring, 2007), while others have responded to workforce shortages (Collyer, 2007). These studies are considered in the context of other means of control or influence by the state or corporate owners in the experience of professional work. The increased presence of clinical governance arguably sits closely alongside managerialism, recognising that clinical leadership is integral to the success of the governance endeavours. However, the role of clinical governance should also be viewed within the wider context of efforts to manage the broader safety and quality agenda and outcomes, incorporating but looking beyond the influence of individuals (Duckett, 2009; Spigelman and Rendalls, 2015).

The emergence of crises that shake the confidence in regulatory arrangements, most notably in relation to medical practitioners in Australia and the United Kingdom (UK), has also been of specific consequence in identifying to the wider community the relevance of regulatory arrangements (Smith, 2002; Faunce and Bolsin, 2004; Harvey and Faunce, 2005). In Australia, however, the influence of the profession has been a less dominant factor in regulatory response to crises. In the most infamous case of regulatory failure, there had been a series of fraudulent representations that were made by Jayant Patel, a surgeon at Bundaberg Hospital in Queensland, in not disclosing prior restrictions on practice. These were revealed via a Google search and the consequences of failings in clinical governance locally (that is, authorising surgery to be undertaken beyond the approved scope of a practitioner) in a stretched environment that resulted in the most serious of patient outcomes (Davies, 2005; Thomas, 2007; Pacey et al, 2010).

But there was conflict between the medical profession and governments across Australia in relation to involvement by some professional membership bodies in two aspects that influenced workforce and its governance – the training of new members of the profession and the assessment of practitioners who had obtained their qualifications overseas. This conflict revolved around arguments about quality and standards and had been prominent in the lead-up to a review by the Productivity Commission. To maintain its engagement with these activities, the Royal Australasian College of Surgeons sought a formal authorisation from the Australian Competition and Consumer Commission. An authorisation was obtained, and the emergent hydra-headed monster of the commonwealth, state and territory governments used this mechanism to voice frustrations through a further review with the competition agency of the related activities of all specialist medical colleges (Lawson et al, 2005). So the impetus for changes in the regulatory arrangements related to health practitioners in Australia was rooted in a productivity domain, but directly characterised by contestation around a (usually) privileged domain of standard setting. As we discuss later in this chapter, the hydra also used its collective authority to pursue wider health workforce agendas through the establishment of the regulatory scheme by including the support of the evolution of a much less recognised and influential profession, that of Aboriginal and Torres Strait Islander health practitioners.

A national solution

The national scheme was designed to bring substantial change to the management of health practitioner regulation in Australia. This change was in terms of both the standardisation of requirements and the centralisation of governance. The standardisation of requirements initially is a measure directed to individual practitioners, but which allows consolidation of data and monitoring. The centralisation of governance is the mechanism that then informs the monitoring of actions that the regulatory agencies undertake in improving public safety and addressing wider health workforce initiatives.

Australia is a federation, with a national government and separate state and territory governments. Each has responsibility for the oversight or delivery of different aspects of public policy or services, which is defined under the written Constitution of 1900. Australia was the location of some of the earliest government or legal recognition of medical practitioners in 1837 in what became the state of Tasmania. What emerged were co-regulatory arrangements, with governments providing a legislative framework and the profession representatives holding majority membership. Across Australia, each of the six states and two territories developed separate legislative frameworks with different health professions regulated, and the same individual practitioners were subject to different expectations and compliance obligations in each location.

This lack of consistency across the country was increasingly becoming a concern to professions and governments. It was part of a set of concerns that the Australian (Commonwealth) government outlined in a major assessment of future economic planning. Known as the Intergenerational Report and part of the 2002-03 Budget papers (Australian Government, 2002), it noted complex factors in ensuring that the future health needs of the community could be delivered and funded. The focus, though, was primarily economic and at a macro level. And, in responding to those challenges, the Australian government instructed the Productivity Commission, the nation's primary economic agency, to undertake a series of reviews to guide national policy. This became a suite of three, focusing on the costs of health technology, the impact of an ageing population and Australia's health workforce. This final investigation sat against a set of challenges that were about more than cost or funding and to a significant extent reflected on the dispersed nature of responsibility. Whether in the field of training, in which universities fall under the jurisdiction of the national government and technical colleges under states and territories, or in the regulation of individual health practitioners, the system was highly fragmented. And this fragmentation made the challenge of national reform formidable indeed.

The Productivity Commission undertook broad consultation and received submissions from a wide range of health professions organisations as well as other stakeholders, including existing regulatory agencies (Productivity Commission, 2005). As indicated earlier, in framing the new regulatory regime, governments needed to be clear and agreed about the risks the scheme should manage in order to protect the public. As previously noted, there had been a long tradition of health practitioner registration in Australia. There had also been some efforts made in seeking to streamline collective endeavours in relation to the health workforce. Some state/territory jurisdictions had already made progress in regulatory reform – with the state of Victoria for instance having moved to a single legislative tool across each of the professions it regulated (Carlton, 2005). As indicated, there had been a series of structural reforms across health policy in 2004 and 2005 in advance of the Productivity Commission's report, including the first national health workforce strategic plan and a health workforce action plan, as well as jurisdictional responses to different failures of regulatory and clinical governance (Rix et al, 2005). This experience of engaging in future planning collaboratively, while responding to crises individually, helped to bolster the desire of governments to seek a truly national solution.

The Productivity Commission recommended three separate bodies – one to register individuals, one to accredit the education and training required to meet registration requirements and another to focus on the workforce endeavour more holistically. Pivoting more on the innovation and productivity agenda, the recommendation for separate national registration and accreditation bodies was endorsed by the Council of Australian Governments – the Prime Minister, Premiers and Chief Ministers in July 2006. They agreed that these two schemes should be established by July 2008 (COAG, 2006). That was, and proved to be, a completely unrealistic timeframe. It was, however, achieved by March 2008 through an intergovernmental agreement that outlined the revised plan. A single scheme was created, a single entity to undertake registration and accreditation functions and profession-specific boards. This agreement demonstrated how much activity had occurred in the preceding 18 months, effectively outlining the blueprint of the future legislation, as well as the variability of legislative processes that would be required through different Parliaments across the land (COAG, 2008).

Birth of the hydra-headed monster

And so the Ministerial Council, our hydra, came into being. The hydra-headed monster is a metaphor that has been applied in exploring complex governance arrangements in different national/multinational contexts (Radin, 1998; Johansson-Nogués, 2014). These two examples share application in a context of reform, one sharing the story of the introduction of a complex piece of legislation in the US (the Government Performance and Results Act) in the 1990s and the other exploring structural changes in representational arrangements of the European Union to the United Nations. In both instances, the authors applied the image of the hydra-headed monster to complex, challenging governance situations in which multiple sources of accountability exist.

Its presence in our story of the national scheme first emerged during the parliamentary inquiry in which the descriptor was tossed in as a response by a public servant in seeking to describe the complexity of the governance arrangements of the scheme – that is, of its multiple boards and accreditation agencies (Legislative Legal and Social Issues Committee, 2014). However, the metaphor is not ideally suited to this use as while these boards are distinctive by professional group, their actions are limited by the legislative framework of the scheme in their actions. However, the application to the governments – and more specifically health ministers – has more suitability, with its description as 'a many-headed sophist, each of whose heads is an argument' (Jackson, 1990: 380). It is also a familiar symbol of power and authority, including in popular culture.[1] But to be clear, the application of the metaphor goes as far as a living hydra-headed monster; the myth of its death and destruction is not adopted – although the vision of states and territories being decapitated (as was the eventual fate of our mythical figure) may be of appeal to those who feel that Australia is over-governed and seek the abolition of the states and territories layer of governments.

A hydra-headed monster

In the iterative preparation and implementation phase, the features of the hydra become clearer. In an account by the senior public official involved in establishing the scheme, we come to learn that ministers effectively engaged in two modes – the heads pivoting towards the external frame with collective effort, and activating the internal argument mode to discuss internal decisions, but with a focus on sustaining the strength derived from a unitary form. Louise Morauta (2011), the senior public servant tasked with the introduction of the scheme, recounts for example that the 'COAG [Council of Australian Governments] mandate and dynamic itself may have motivated Ministers to reach agreement.... Ministers may have felt that if they could not reach agreement, somebody else might want to do that for them'. It is valuable to consider these motivations when we move to consider the accountability arrangements of the scheme as they pertain to this ministerial agglomeration.

As noted earlier, the existing constitution responsibility for health practitioner regulation sat with state and territory governments. But there had over time been increasing endeavours by governments in collaboration to identify national solutions, often with the enticement of specific funding from the Commonwealth, which has the superior income-raising capacity (Brumby and Galligan, 2015). So, it was into this environment that the work began in earnest.

Governance and accountability arrangements – accountability in the public interest

With the commitment of six state, two territory and a federal government through the intergovernmental agreement, the process of collective governance arrangements began. In doing so, they committed to an enduring endeavour in which they would be held together and constrained by the form that was adopted. The pursuit of national arrangements for the national registration and accreditation of the health professions was one of a number grouped under the 'Seamless National Economy' banner and featured as one of the successful productivity reforms achieved under this initiative (COAG Reform Council, 2012) .

Yet, the legislative and governance arrangements even for other new regulatory bodies were not as distinctive as those for the bodies established to oversee the registration of health professionals and the accreditation of educational qualifications leading to registrations. A national law model was adopted, which meant that consistent legislation was required to be approved by each state and territory Parliament in order to deliver an outcome. This was consistent, but not the same, as small differences were required to be accommodated, including in the Australian Capital Territory – ensuring that its legislation was compatible with the provisions of its human rights framework. With the structure of the scheme as defined, its objectives established the detailed work that remained to be addressed.

The core artefact at this stage of regulatory endeavour was the substantial Regulatory Impact Statement. This work was presented to the ministerial hydra by the committee of health officials commissioned to complete the task, and included the reassurance that it had been approved as a 'COAG decision-making Regulatory Impact Statement' by the Office of Best Practice Regulation in the Australian Government Department of Finance and Deregulation (Australian Health Ministers' Advisory Council, 2009). It serves as a testament to the challenges of the clean-slate approach adopted in the establishment of the new scheme. As Chamberlain (2016: 13) notes, in the environment of high modernity, governments are judged (in) 'their ability to manage risk that [the] state legitimises its governing activities', reflecting also the commentary of Haines (2011) discussed earlier in the Australian setting. It is this document that most clearly identifies exactly the scope of protection of the public that is envisaged. Across each profession, 13 'risk' activities were reviewed and assessed, incorporating those relating to technical skills or practices, but also those where boundary issues may be more present. This actuarial-style assessment was undertaken not solely on those professions that were regulated previously in all jurisdictions, but also on those that were defined as partially regulated – not regulated in all jurisdictions. One of these was Aboriginal and Torres Strait Islander health practitioners, registered only in the Northern Territory. As noted earlier in this chapter, there is a significant gap in life expectancy between Aboriginal and Torres Strait Islander and other Australians. The capacity to address an area of defined socio-political risk through regulation sat within a wider reform agenda (Mason, 2013).

Returning to a theme previously discussed, this scenario represents the affirmation of the state (the governments across Australia) in actively designing the new regulatory regime in a very intentional way to concurrently address public safety and productivity/service delivery priorities – neither of which is fixed and both of which have the capacity to be informed by experience. An important site of tension between the professions and our hydra-headed monster is also highlighted in the discussion within the Regulatory Impact Statement over the responsibility for making determinations relating to accreditation. This was a repeated site of tension, outlined in submissions to the Productivity Commission (2005) – with a Senate Committee inquiry reporting that the independence of accreditation processes under the scheme was perhaps the major issue raised (Senate Community Affairs Committee, 2009). In 2016, following an independent review of the scheme, further work reviewed the range of accreditation arrangements (independent bodies and created adjunct bodies) to assess how the public interest is, or should be, addressed within the wider context of the scheme (Australian Health Ministers' Advisory Council, 2014; COAG Health Council/Australian Health Workforce Ministerial Council, 2015).

In order for the community to have confidence that this newly established regulatory framework is undertaking its activities with both the protection of the public and the wider public interest considered, the provision of information (and of outcomes) about its activities need to be available, clear and targeted and evidence-based (Bismark et al, 2015). While there are a range of audiences that may have different expectations and needs to be satisfied in this regard, only obligations to the hydra are being considered here, as the connecting entity to the state, embodying the public as democratically elected governments. The primary obligation in relation to reporting is to the hydra's individual heads, by way of annual reports presented to each health minister, who is then required to have these tabled in each Parliament. In a previous study, we identified that between 2010 and 2015, this requirement had been met (Pacey et al, 2017). Legislation has also been passed in each state and territory, which has endorsed the scope for those Parliaments to undertake their own inquiries on the scheme. An inquiry has been held by a parliamentary committee in Victoria (Legislative Legal and Social Issues Committee, 2014), as well as in the Australian Parliament (Senate Community Affairs Committee, 2010; Senate Finance and Public Administration References Committee, 2011).

But, it is at this juncture that the hydra's unitary form becomes problematic as any individual minister responding to the Parliament in the jurisdiction in which they hold office, does not hold a mandate to guarantee change as a member of a combined entity. Even as a collective entity, the status of a Ministerial Council remains somewhat shrouded in mystery (Carney, 2006; Kildea and Lynch, 2011). As no individual minister has the authority to institute change to the national scheme unilaterally, they would be unlikely to purport to be able to do so. This is not to suggest that the relationship has been without tensions as the hydra moved into operational mode over the scheme. As discussed previously, ministers demonstrated the capacity to compromise, including in accepting some elements of difference in the design of the scheme (Morauta, 2011). In 2015, the hydra publicly signalled a lack of agreement on a key question relating to the incorporation of an additional professional group in the scheme. At a meeting in late 2015, a communiqué indicated that one jurisdiction 'reserved its right' to participate and the Commonwealth had dissented (COAG Health Council, 2015). Within the space of a year, however, all contentious matters had been resolved and agreement for the registration of paramedics across all states and territories was approved for inclusion in the scheme, at the same meeting where there was agreement that social workers would not be incorporated (COAG Health Council, 2016). The status then of registered (and recognised) professions by the hydra in this way has continued to affirm their gatekeeper status, and been able to define a public interest that may be influenced at different time points more significantly by risks that are more actuarial or socio-political in concern.

Conclusion

Australia's system of health workforce governance is unique. It has a single national system, with a single legislative tool, and is operationalised through a unified organisation. This is differentiated from the UK with multiple legislation and organisations, New Zealand with a single legislative tool and multiple profession-specific organisations, and the US with governance being predominantly undertaken at a state level. It is too early to conclude whether the national scheme, through its constituent parts of the Australian Health Practitioner Regulation Agency and the national boards, is successful in colonising the regulatory space in a way that diminishes the power of the Ministerial Council, the hydra-headed monster.

Will the registration and accreditation functions merge over time or separate as had been initially planned? The independent review of the accreditation organisations will begin to illuminate the pathway for our mythical creature – perhaps deviating and concentrating its efforts towards those components that more closely align the levers of workforce planning. In this way, it remains the scenario in Australia that the entities within the national scheme – currently 14 profession-specific boards and the Australian Health Practitioner Regulation Agency – are assigned specific functions reflecting the objectives of the establishing legislation. As highlighted in this study, these objectives maintain the presence of the state (all state, territory and federal governments) as the dominant influence beyond the professions in the sphere of health workforce regulation and governance. As this chapter has outlined, this outcome has emerged from a commitment to the protection of the public, while also being aware of broader policy concerns regarding the availability of suitability qualified health practitioners. Although regulatory failures informed the timing of the scheme's development and introduction, the key impetus reflected a deliberative response to address existing workforce challenges, including some that were sites of contestation between the medical profession in particular and the state. The position of the state has now been secured. Under the new national regulatory arrangements the hydra-headed monster, the national Ministerial Council, is the ultimate authority in the management of actuarial and socio-political risks.

Note

[1.] 'Hydra' is also well known in popular culture to fans of the *Marvel* comic series, featuring in the movie and television adaptation of the comic books of an earlier era. The decidedly evil intent of that organisation is not suggested in our appropriation of the mythical figure.

Acknowledgement

The authors wish to acknowledge the constructive feedback received from colleagues in a Research Committee of Professional Groups session at the third International Sociological Association Forum of Sociology in Vienna in July 2016, at which some of the elements included in this chapter were presented.

References

Australian Government (2002) *Intergenerational Report 2002-2003*, Canberra: Commonwealth of Australia, http://www.treasury.gov.au/contentitem.asp?ContentID=378&NavID=

Australian Health Ministers' Advisory Council (2009) *Regulatory Impact Statement for the Decision to Implement the Health Practitioner Regulation National Law: Report from the Governance Committee of the National Registration and Accreditation Implementation Project*, reference no. 10513, Canberra, Australia: Office of Best Practice Regulation.

Australian Health Ministers' Advisory Council (2014) *Independent Review of the National Registration and Accreditation Scheme for Health Professionals*, Adelaide, Australia: COAG Health Council, www.coaghealthcouncil.gov.au/Projects/Independent-Review-of-NRAS-finalised/ArtMID/524/ArticleID/64/Consultation-Paper-August-2014-Review-of-the-National-Registration-and-Accreditation-Scheme-for-health-professionals

Australian Health Practitioner Regulation Agency (2016) *AHPRA June 2016 Newsletter*, www.ahpra.gov.au/Publications/AHPRA-newsletter/June-2016.aspx

Bismark, M., Fletcher, M., Spittal, M. and Studdert, D. (2015) 'A step towards evidence-based regulation of health practitioners', *Australian Health Review* 39(4): 483-5.

Brumby, J. and Galligan, B. (2015) 'The federalism debate', *Australian Journal of Public Administration* 74(1): 82-92.

Carlton, A.-L. (2005) 'National models for regulation of the health professions', *Law in Context* 23(2): 21-51.

Carney, G. (2006) *The Constitutional Systems of the Australian States and Territories*, Cambridge: Cambridge University Press.

Chamberlain, J. M. (2013) *The Sociology of Medical Regulation: An Introduction*, London: Springer.

Chamberlain, J. M. (2016) 'An introduction to medicine, risk, discourse and power', in Chamberlain, J. M. (ed) *Medicine, Risk, Discourse and Power*, London: Taylor & Francis.

COAG (Council of Australian Governments) (2006) *Council of Australian Governments Meeting: 14 July 2006: Communique*, Canberra, Australia: COAG, http://ncp.ncc.gov.au/docs/Council%20of%20 Australian%20Governments%20Meeting%20-%2014%20July%20 2006.pdf

COAG (2008) *Intergovernmental Agreement for a National Registration and Accreditation Scheme for the Health Professions*, Canberra, Australia: COAG, www.ahpra.gov.au/documents/default.aspx?record=WD1 0%2f36&dbid=AP&chksum=NwgooGtzxb6JjNBIEP9Lhg%3d%3d

COAG Health Council (2015) *COAG Health Council Communique: 6 November 2015*, Adelaide: COAG Health Council, www. coaghealthcouncil.gov.au/Announcements/ArtMID/527/ ArticleID/74/CHC-Communique-6-November-2015

COAG Health Council (2016) *COAG Health Council Communique: 7 October 2016* Adelaide: COAG Health Council, www. coaghealthcouncil.gov.au/Announcements/ArtMID/527/ ArticleID/93/7-October-2016-COAG-Health-Council- Communique

COAG Health Council/Australian Health Workforce Ministerial Council (2015) *Communique: The Independent Review of the National Registration and Accreditation Scheme for Health Professions*, Adelaide: COAG Health Council, www.coaghealthcouncil.gov.au/Portals/0/ The%20Independent%20Review%20of%20the%20National%20 Registration%20and%20Accreditation%20Scheme%20for%20 Health%20Professions.pdf

COAG Reform Council (2012) *Seamless National Economy: Report on Performance – Report to the Council of Australian Governments (3rd Annual Report)*, Sydney: COAG Reform Council.

Collyer, F. (2007) 'A sociological approach to workforce shortages: findings of a qualitative study in Australian hospitals', *Health Sociology Review* 16(3-4): 248-62.

Davies, G. (2005) *Queensland Public Hospitals Commission of Inquiry*, Brisbane, Australia: Queensland Government.

Duckett, S. (2009) 'Transforming clinical governance in Queensland health', in Healy, J. and Dugdale, P. (eds) *Patient Safety First: Responsive Regulation in Health Care*, Sydney: Allen & Unwin.

Faunce, T. A. and Bolsin, S. N. C. (2004) 'Three Australian whistleblowing sagas: lessons for internal and external regulation', *Medical Journal of Australia* 181(1): 44-7.

Haines, F. (2011) *The Paradox of Regulation: What Regulation Can Achieve and What it Cannot*, Cheltenham: Edward Elgar.

Harvey, K. and Faunce, T. (2005) 'A critical analysis of overseas-trained doctor (otd) factors in the Bundaberg Base Hospital Surgical Inquiry', *Law in Context* 23(2): 73-91.

Healy, J. (2011) *Improving Health Care Safety and Quality: Reluctant Regulators*, Farnham: Ashgate.

Healy, J. and Braithwaite, J. (2006) 'Designing safer health care through responsive regulation', *Medical Journal of Australia* 184(10): S56-S59.

Jackson, R. (1990) 'Socrates' Iolaos: myth and eristic in Plato's Euthydemus', *The Classical Quarterly* 40(2): 378-95.

Johansson-Nogués, E. (2014) 'The European Union's external representation after Lisbon: from "hydra-headed" to "octopus"?', *EUI-RSCAS Working Papers*, http://cadmus.eui.eu/bitstream/handle/1814/29921/RSCAS_2014_15.pdf

Kildea, P. and Lynch, A. (2011) 'Entrenching "cooperative federalism": is it time to formalise COAG's place in the Australian federation?', *Federal Law Review* 39(1): 103-29.

Kohn, L. T., Corrigan, J. and Donaldson, M. S. (2000) *To Err Is Human: Building a Safer Health System*, Washington, DC: National Academies Press.

Kuhlmann, E. and Larsen, C. (2015) 'Why we need multi-level health workforce governance: case studies from nursing and medicine in Germany', *Health Policy*, 119(2): 1636-44.

Kuhlmann, E. and Saks, M. (2008) 'Changing patterns of health professional governance', in Kuhlmann, E. and Saks, M. (eds) *Rethinking Professional Governance: International Directions in Healthcare*, Bristol: Policy Press.

Lawson, K. A., Gregory, A. T. and van der Weyden, M. B. (2005) 'The medical colleges in Australia: besieged but bearing up', *Medical Journal of Australia* 183(11/12): 646-51.

Legislative Legal and Social Issues Committee (2014) *Inquiry into the Performance of the Australian Health Practitioner Regulation Agency*, Melbourne, Australia: Parliament of Victoria.

Liljegren, A. and Saks, M. (2016) *Professions and Metaphors: Understanding Professions in Society*, London: Routledge.

Mason, J. (2013) *Review of Australian Government Health Workforce Programs*, https://www.health.gov.au/internet/main/publishing. nsf/Content/D26858F4B68834EACA257BF0001A8DDC/$File/Review%20of%20Health%20Workforce%20programs.pdf

Morauta, L. (2011) 'Implementing a COAG reform using the national law model: Australia's National Registration and Accreditation Scheme for Health Practitioners', *Australian Journal of Public Administration* 70(1): 75–83.

Negin, J., Rozea, A., Cloyd, B. and Martiniuk, A. L. (2013) 'Foreign-born health workers in Australia: an analysis of census data', *Human Resources for Health* 11(1): 69–78.

Pacey, F., Short, S. and Harley, K. (2010) 'The Patel case and its consequences for health workforce governance in Australia - rapid response', *British Medical Journal* 341, www.bmj.com/content/341/bmj.c3646/rapid-responses

Pacey, F., Smith-Merry, J., Gillespie, J. and Short, S. (2017) 'National health workforce regulation: contextualising the Australian scheme', *International Journal of Health Governance* 22(1): 5–14.

Palmer, G. and Short, S. (2014) *Health Care and Public Policy: An Australian Analysis*, South Yarra, Australia: Palgrave Macmillan.

Productivity Commission (2005) *Australia's Health Workforce*, Canberra, Australia: Commonwealth of Australia.

Radin, B. A. (1998) 'The Government Performance and Results Act (GPRA): hydra-headed monster or flexible management tool?', *Public Administration Review* 58(4): 307–16.

Rix, M., Owen, A. and Eagar, K. (2005) '(Re)form with substance? Restructuring and governance in the Australian health system 2004/05', *Australia and New Zealand Health Policy* 2(1): 19–27.

Rogers, S. (2004) 'Culling bad apples, blowing whistles and the Health Practitioners Competence Assurance Act 2003 (NZ)', *Journal of Law and Medicine* 12(1): 119–33.

Saks, M. (2015) *The Professions, State and the Market: Medicine in Britain, the United States and Russia*, London: Routledge.

Salter, B (2003) 'Patients and doctors: reformulating the UK health policy community?', *Social Science and Medicine* 57(5): 927–36.

Senate Community Affairs Committee, Parliament of Australia (2009) *National Accreditation Scheme for Doctors and Other Health Workers*, Canberra, Australia: Parliament of Australia.

Senate Community Affairs Committee, Parliament of Australia (2010) *Health Practitioner Regulation (Consequential Amendment) Bill 2010 [Provisions]*, Canberra, Australia: Parliament of Australia.

Senate Finance and Public Administration References Committee, Parliament of Australia (2011) *The Administration of Health Practitioner Registration by the Australian Health Practitioner Regulation Agency (AHPRA)*, Canberra, Australia: Parliament of Australia.

Smith, D. (2002) 'Not by error – but by design: Harold Shipman and the regulatory crisis for health care', *Public Policy and Administration* 17(4): 55-74.

Spigelman, A. D. and Rendalls, S. (2015) 'Clinical governance in Australia', *Clinical Governance: An International Journal* 20(2): 56-73.

Thomas, H. (2007) *Sick to Death: A Manipulative Surgeon and a Health System in Crisis – A Disaster Waiting to Happen*, Sydney, Australia: Allen & Unwin.

Waring, J. (2007) 'Adaptive regulation or governmentality: patient safety and the changing regulation of medicine', *Sociology of Health and Illness* 29(2): 163-79.

World Health Organization (2017) '*Health systems – stewardship*', www.who.int/healthsystems/stewardship/en/

Health complaints entities in Australia and New Zealand: serving the public interest?

Jennifer Morris, Jennifer Moore and Marie Bismark

Introduction

This chapter discusses health complaints entities in Australia and New Zealand. Health complaints entities are responsible for receiving and resolving patients' complaints about the quality of health care services.[1] In many jurisdictions, such as Australia (Bismark et al, 2013), New Zealand (Dew and Roorda, 2001), Scandinavia (Rosenthal, 1992), the United Kingdom (UK) (Nettleton and Harding, 1994; Chamberlain, 2013) and the United States (Dauer, 2011), there has been sustained interest in patients' complaints since the 1990s. While research has typically focused on formal complaints, it is recognised that these represent only a small fraction of patients' concerns about their care (Beaupert et al, 2014).

Complaints from patients have attracted growing interest from policy makers and professional organisations, largely because of the social movement promoting patients' rights in health care. Factors such as media coverage of medical injuries, the establishment of patient advocacy groups and the increasing availability of information, have heightened health care users' awareness of patient safety issues, and increased the demand for accountability. In addition to accountability, research suggests that patients[2] who raise concerns about care often seek remedies such as apologies, explanations, and corrective action to prevent harm to future patients (Bismark et al, 2011; Moore and Mello, 2017; Moore et al, 2017). Health complaints entities may provide such remedies. In doing so, health complaints entities have the potential to serve the public interest, particularly with respect to public health and safety, open justice and economic benefits. In this chapter, we explore the extent to which health complaints entities in Australia and New Zealand are maximising their potential to serve the public interest.

While there are variations between health care complaints processes and outcomes depending on the jurisdiction, a similarity that crosses jurisdictional boundaries is that many countries have transitioned from self-regulation to greater external oversight by the state (Beaupert et al, 2014). Health complaints entities represent one regulatory strategy, working alongside clinical governance and professional self-regulation. By encompassing broader concerns and remedies than medical malpractice litigation (Bismark et al, 2011), health complaints entities are now the main avenues for patients and their families who want action to address problems relating to their treatment. Health complaints entities have been likened to patient ombudsman systems that operate in jurisdictions such as Austria, Finland, Greece, Israel, Norway and the UK (Fallberg and MacKenney, 2003; Beaupert et al, 2014). The independent ombudsman is tasked with representing the public's interest by investigating complaints against public sector bodies.

This chapter comprises six further sections. First, we describe the establishment of health complaints entities in Australia and New Zealand. Second, we outline the scope, powers, aims and functions of these entities. Third, we explain the processes by which they resolve patients' complaints. Fourth, we analyse the ways in which they serve the public interest. Fifth, we identify several emerging challenges and opportunities for health complaints entities. Finally we conclude the chapter.

Establishment of health complaints entities

Health complaints entities are statutory organisations that receive, and seek to resolve, complaints from the public regarding health care services. Such entities were established in Australia and New Zealand in the late 1980s and the 1990s. They have been in continuous operation since that time, although their powers and processes have evolved.

In New Zealand, a single health complaints entity, the Health and Disability Commissioner (HDC), serves the entire country. The HDC was created by the Health and Disability Commissioner Act, which was enacted in October 1994. The first Commissioner, Robyn Stent, was appointed in December 1994. At the time of writing, the Australian health complaints entities include the:

- Health and Community Services Complaints Commission (Northern Territory);
- Health and Community Services Complaints Commissioner (South Australia);

- Health and Disability Services Complaints Office (Western Australia);
- Health Care Complaints Commission (New South Wales);
- Health Complaints Commissioner (Tasmania);
- Health Complaints Commissioner (Victoria);
- Health Services Commissioner (Australian Capital Territory);
- Office of the Health Ombudsman (Queensland).

These health complaints entities were established after the Australian government introduced the Medicare Agreements Act 1992, which stated that the eight states and two mainland territories must establish and maintain health complaints bodies that were independent of government. Each health complaints entity was created by state or territory legislation. For example, the New South Wales Health Care Complaints Commission was established under the Health Care Complaints Act 1993 and the Victorian Office of the Health Services Commissioner was created under the Health Services (Conciliation and Review) Act 1987, with its powers revised under the Health Complaints Act 2016.

The introduction of health complaints entities occurred as two significant shifts in attitudes and awareness around health care gathered momentum in many countries. First, a landmark study of adverse events revealed the extent of preventable harm being experienced by patients in hospitals (Brennan et al, 1991). Second, a movement focused on patients' rights, and patient empowerment, was beginning to shift attitudes, power dynamics and expectations. In New Zealand, a third major event prompted the creation of the HDC – the *Report of the Cervical Cancer Inquiry*. The report is often referred to as the Cartwright Report, in reference to Judge Silvia Cartwright, who led the inquiry (Cartwright, 1988). The inquiry uncovered a multitude of issues with the practices of Associate Professor Herbert Green at New Zealand's National Women's Hospital, including unconsented and unauthorised research, and deliberate under-treatment of cervical cancer. Judge Cartwright made many recommendations, including the introduction of both an independent complaints commissioner and a code of patients' rights. The implementation of these recommendations was supported by the newly created Health and Disability Commissioner Act 1994.

The recommendation that led New Zealand to introduce a code of patients' rights came to fruition via the Code of Health and Disability Services Consumers' Rights ('the Code'), which became law in 1996. The full text of the Code (which includes 10 rights) is available on the HDC website (Health and Disability Commissioner, 2016). The Code, and the complaints mechanisms under the New Zealand Health and Disability Commissioner Act, has since become 'the primary vehicle for dealing with complaints about the quality of care' (Health and Disability Commissioner, 2016).

Like New Zealand, Australia has also recognised a core set of patients' rights, enshrined in the Australian Charter of Healthcare Rights ('the Charter') (Australian Commission on Safety and Quality in Healthcare, 2008). A key difference between the New Zealand Code and Australian Charter concerns their enforceability. The New Zealand version provides a codified benchmark against which the health complaints entity assesses complaints for potential breaches. Providers who infringe a patient's rights can be held to account for their actions (Wall, 2016). In contrast, the Australian Charter 'allows patients, consumers, families, carers and service providers to have a common understanding of the rights of people receiving healthcare' (Australian Commission on Safety and Quality in Healthcare, 2008). The Australian Charter is effectively a guide only. It is not specifically enforceable, and it is not linked to the powers of the health complaints entities. In the next section, we explore health complaints entities' powers in more detail.

Scope, powers, aims and functions

As outlined in the previous section, each health complaints entity is established by a statute, which describes its scope, powers, aims and functions. The scope of some health complaints entities includes services other than health care, such as disability or community services. However, this chapter will only consider their responsibilities in the health care sector.

A series of scandals and public inquiries have led to governments changing certain features of health complaints entities, usually in favour of stronger and broader-reaching powers. Their specific processes and powers vary between jurisdictions, but their overarching purpose and features remain broadly comparable. For example, all health complaints entities operate independently of government, health care services and health practitioners. Two core aims are common across health complaints entities. First, they are charged with promoting effective complaints handling by receiving, assessing, investigating and resolving complaints from patients about health care services. Second, they aim to inform health care improvement by identifying, reporting on and/ or advocating for change on the basis of complaints about health care services.

Health complaints entities' main functions map on to their aims, and are captured by the New Zealand HDC's mission, which is to 'independently uphold consumer rights by promotion and protection, resolving complaints, service monitoring, advocacy and education' (Health and Disability Commissioner, 2014). The first core function of health complaints entities is to provide a direct-service case-based complaints management service to the public. In this role, they assist members of the public (typically users of health care services or their family or friends) to make complaints about their health care experiences, have those complaints heard and (where possible) achieve satisfactory resolution of those complaints. In this role, health complaints entities serve as impartial third parties, working together with members of the public and health care providers in resolving complaints.

To achieve their direct-service function, health complaints entities utilise a variety of complaint resolution approaches, ranging from brief informal communication to prolonged dispute resolution. Common approaches include facilitating communication between complainants and services or practitioners, seeking clarification, explanation or apology for complainants, and more structured alternative dispute resolution such as conciliation and mediation. In serious cases, commissioners may act as gatekeepers to disciplinary proceedings. This direct-service role is essentially reactive, responding to negative experiences of health care after they occur. At present, this reactive, direct-service role comprises the bulk of the work undertaken by health complaints entities.

The second main function of health complaints entities involves educating the public, practitioners, health services and others about ways to improve health care quality and safety. Through their role as recipients of complaints, health complaints entities gather a wealth of knowledge, both anecdotal and empirical, about recurring problems with the safety and quality of care provided in their jurisdictions. For example, they may become aware of particular health practitioners or services that attract a disproportionate number of complaints, or aspects of care that are commonly complained about. Their quality improvement role allows health complaints entities to disseminate lessons learned through one or more individual complaints, potentially mitigating or preventing future negative experiences of health care. According to former New Zealand Health and Disability Commissioner, Professor Paterson, complaints may be used as a 'window of opportunity' to improve health care (Paterson, 2002). As will be discussed later in this chapter, the degree to which health complaints entities engage in this role is limited and varies by jurisdiction, reflecting differences in statutory powers, resourcing, legal issues and cultural norms.

Importantly, health complaints entities provide an option for people wishing to make a complaint about a practitioner who is not a member of a registered profession, and who is therefore beyond the reach of any health practitioner regulator. Health workforce regulators (for instance, the Medical Board of Australia) only have jurisdiction over individuals who are students or members of one of the registered professions included in their remits, or who apply to be or falsely claim to be members of these professions. In addition, they can only receive complaints about individual practitioners, as opposed to health services or institutions. Thus, regulators cannot ensure adequate public protection from unsafe health services, or people practising in professions over which regulators do not have jurisdiction. By contrast, health complaints entities have the power to receive complaints about individuals or entities offering or providing any type of health service, including professions not covered by health workforce regulators.

It is also important to note the role of health complaints entities in the context of other legal avenues available to compensate harmed patients in the relevant jurisdictions. Civil proceedings (rather than disciplinary proceedings) are required if a New Zealand patient is to receive damages for a breach of the Code (for example, due to discrimination). However, in New Zealand, an injured patient cannot seek compensatory damages for a 'personal injury' (including medical injury) that falls within the scope of New Zealand's national no-fault accident compensation scheme, the Accident Compensation Corporation (ACC). In New Zealand, ACC replaced the former torts system with a government-funded scheme for compensating people with personal injuries. Therefore, even when negligent treatment causes injury and constitutes a breach of the Code, a claim for compensatory damages is precluded by law.

By contrast, Australian patients who experience medical injuries may seek compensation through civil litigation, or, if permanently disabled as a result, may seek funding for disability support services from the National Disability Insurance Scheme. The National Disability Insurance Scheme is designed to complement, not replace, existing compensation claims. It does not preclude recovery of compensation elsewhere – as, for instance, for medical negligence. However, the prior receipt of compensation from other sources may reduce entitlements from the National Disability Insurance Scheme (Madden, 2016). While the civil litigation option is available, Dauer (2011) has claimed that Australia has 'curbed' malpractice litigation by offering parallel commission-based procedures. Table 12.1 compares the functions of health complaints entities with those of two other agencies that handle medico-legal matters in Australia: civil courts and the Medical Board of Australia.

It is important to note that the above-described avenues are not necessarily mutually exclusive. Injured patients who seek non-monetary and monetary remedies may lodge a complaint to a health complaints

Table 12.1: Focus, functions and remedies of key entities with responsibility for medico-legal matters in Australia

	Health complaints entities	Civil courts	Medical Board of Australia
Jurisdictional focus	Low-quality care Patient dissatisfaction with care or services	Substandard care causing patient harm	Professional misconduct or unprofessional conduct Performance or competence falling below accepted standards Substance misuse or impairment affecting practice
Cases handled	Complaints from the public	Negligence claims	Matters concerning the conduct, performance or health of doctors
Procedures used	Early resolution Conciliation Investigation	Out-of-court negotiation Alternative forms of dispute resolution (for example, mediation or arbitration) Trials before judges	Review of the doctor's competence or health status Investigation Disciplinary action
Remedies	Communication (for instance, facilitate apology or explanation) Restoration (for example, facilitate provision of further treatment, fee forgiveness or monetary settlement) Correction (for instance, recommend system change)	Monetary damages	Correction (for example, a requirement that the practitioner undergoes education, rehabilitation or monitoring) Sanction (for instance, suspension or the revocation of practising rights)

entity, and also file a claim with ACC (in New Zealand) or in the civil courts (in Australia), in pursuit of those respective aims.

Processes for health complaints

Health complaints entities can receive complaints from a variety of sources. These include patients, someone making a complaint on a patient's behalf, advocates and any other member of the public. Complaints can be made about any health service, including individual practitioners or organisations (such as a clinic or hospital). Complaints can be about clinical or non-clinical matters. Some common issues raised in complaints include access to a service, administrative matters, privacy and confidentiality, treatment or diagnosis, communication, disrespect, discrimination and costs (Paterson, 2015; Paterson and Manning, 2017). The main activity of the health complaints entity is to provide dispute resolution and conciliation processes to reach a mutually agreeable resolution to the complaint.

Health complaints entities encourage potential complainants, where possible, to raise their concerns with the service provider before lodging a complaint with the health complaints entity. For those who do wish to complain to a health complaints entity, the service is free of charge, does not require the involvement of a lawyer and is intended to be readily accessible. However, several health complaints entities still require that complaints be made in writing. This can serve as a barrier to some patients, including those with low education, low literacy or whose primary language is not English.

Once received, each complaint is triaged. This includes assessing whether it falls within the health complaints entity's jurisdiction, whether it would be better managed by another agency (for example, the police) and whether it is suitable for low-level resolution, or if more formal investigation or assessment is required. Each health complaints entity communicates closely with health practitioner boards, such as the Medical Board of Australia and the Medical Council of New Zealand. Health complaints entities may pass on a complaint to the relevant board if it raises issues or risks that warrant regulatory consideration. However, former New Zealand Health and Disability Commissioner, Professor Paterson, maintained that the emphasis of health complaints entities' processes should be on 'learning not lynching' and 'resolution not retribution' (Paterson, 2008).

If a complaint remains in the hands of the health complaints entity, the health care provider that is the subject of the complaint is provided with an opportunity to respond. Under the New Zealand Health and

Disability Commissioner Act 1994, the Commissioner has the power to obtain any information relevant to an investigation. By contrast, in Australia, participation in health complaints entities' processes is voluntary, and providers may choose not to respond or be involved. This is a significant limitation of the Australian health complaints entity system. If a registered practitioner chooses not to engage with the health complaints entity's process, and there are concerns about patient safety, the matter may be referred to their registration board. However, unregistered practitioners and institutions or services cannot be held to account in the same way. As a result, health complaints entities have been criticised for being 'paper tigers' against uncooperative and unregistered practitioners and services (Skegg, 2011). While the health complaints entity may be able to refer some cases to other entities for court action (including the police or the Australian Competition and Consumer Commission), such action is not common. During her time in the position, former Victorian Health Services Commissioner, Dr Beth Wilson, campaigned for a system of 'negative licensing', whereby problematic but unregistered individuals can be banned from offering or providing any kind of health service, whether that type of health service is usually regulated or not. When the Health Complaints Act 2016 was enacted, this power was finally granted to the newly-renamed Victorian Health Complaints Commissioner, who can now impose 'prohibition orders' on individuals and health services.

If the provider chooses to engage with the complaints process, the health complaints entity staff will usually attempt to facilitate a mutually agreeable resolution to the complaint. Examples of outcomes include answers to questions about what happened, apology, remedial treatment, refund, compensation or an explanation of what has been done to prevent recurrences. This may be done formally or informally, including through phone calls, letters or face-to-face meetings. Formal conciliation has recognised status under law, and information shared during formal conciliation proceedings is often subject to legal privilege, and cannot be used against an individual or service in legal proceedings. At any stage, the complainant (and, in Australia, the provider) can choose to withdraw from involvement in health complaints entities' processes. In more serious cases, health complaints entities may initiate a formal investigation and some have the power to refer a matter for consideration of disciplinary charges.

In Australia and New Zealand the model of alternative dispute resolution utilised by health complaints entities is not unique to the context of health care complaints. Similar approaches are also used in certain forms of legal disputes (such as family law matters), in restorative justice approaches to crime, in the processes of various Parliament-appointed ombudsmen and in culturally adaptive approaches to criminal proceedings involving indigenous offenders.

The interface with the public interest

Any consideration of whether health complaints entities serve the public interest requires a shared understanding of what is meant by 'the public interest'. In its broadest sense, the public interest refers to the wellbeing of the general public and is often considered to be synonymous with 'the common good'. The Australian Law Reform Commission (2014) has proposed a non-exhaustive list of public interest matters, which includes three of particular relevance to the role of health complaints entities: public health and safety, economic prosperity and open justice.

Public health and safety

Public health is optimised when populations achieve and maintain the best possible health and wellbeing for all, within the limits of current knowledge, technology and resources. Elements that contribute to this domain include both the quality of the health service and broader social determinants of health, including health literacy, social services, human rights and social equality. Public safety is achieved when risks of harm are identified early, and prevented or mitigated. The establishment of health complaints entities offers significant potential benefits for public health and safety. These benefits can be conceptualised as ripples spreading out from the patient and provider involved in any particular, individual complaint.

The most immediate potential health and safety benefits are to the thousands of complainants who interact with health complaints entities every year. Patients and those close to them may often find it intimidating, uncomfortable or confronting to complain directly to an individual or organisation that provides health services. These concerns are heightened in certain circumstances – such as where a service operates in a small community, where there are few similar services (for example, a particular type of specialist) or where a person is vulnerable due to factors such age, education, language, culture or disability. Through complaint resolution services offered by health complaints entities, patients' health and safety may be supported through several means. These include:

- restoring a therapeutic relationship that may facilitate future care;
- access to remedial health services for harm they have suffered; and/or
- receiving an explanation about their condition, the treatment they received and any adverse consequences.

However, as we discuss in the 'challenges and opportunities' section of this chapter, the potential benefits for individual complainants are not always fully realised.

The next wave of public health and safety benefits encompasses health care providers who are involved with health complaints entities' processes. As a result of the complaint resolution process, providers may become aware of deficiencies in their own skills, processes or practices that could be remediated for the benefit of future patients. Practitioners and services may be more inclined to engage in open, honest dialogue about the complaint when they are protected by legal privilege in conciliation proceedings.

Health complaints entities have documented successes facilitating complaint-driven learning, changes and improvements at the level of individual practitioners and services (Paterson, 2008). Indeed, one of the most common requests made by complainants is to receive an explanation of what will be done in the future to prevent recurrence of the issue (Bismark et al, 2011; Moore and Mello, 2017; Moore et al, 2017). Many practitioners and services appear to capitalise on the opportunity to improve in response to a complaint to a health complaints entity. For example, they may respond through a change in information provided, policy, process, language or attitude. However, one current limitation of health complaints entities is that most do not have the power to enforce compliance with agreements or promises arising from the complaints-handling process. Therefore, there is no guarantee that promises made about service improvements will be followed through, and health complaints entities' reports of complaints outcomes do not account for the degree to which this actually occurs.

Finally, beyond the parties immediately involved, health complaints entities could also promote public health and safety by educating other providers about patterns of concern, and potential solutions, identified by particular complaints. The day-to-day work of health complaints entities generates a lot of valuable information that could be used to support widespread quality and safety improvement in Australia and New Zealand. This information could be used to detect recurring risks, issues and incidents of harm, as well as the factors that contribute to them, and the ways in which they might be prevented or reduced. For example, in New Zealand, the HDC occasionally publishes findings and recommendations regarding specific cases, including resulting recommendations. Through such activities, health complaints entities could widely disseminate information regarding the lessons learned from complaints, and any improvement strategies developed as a result. Health complaints entities also have the capacity to shed light on systemic problems in health care, such as a high failure rate for certain medical devices.

However, limited analysis of complaints data hampers the ability of health complaints entities to improve public health and safety at a systems level (Bismark and Studdert, 2010). In addition, in Australia, public communication about particular cases is exceptionally rare. In many jurisdictions and circumstances it is disallowed by legislation, or the legality of such public disclosure is uncertain. This is a substantial missed opportunity, because the same lessons must be learned repeatedly by a succession of practitioners, services and institutions. Furthermore, information about effective solutions is not disseminated widely, hampering more widespread progress towards safer, higher-quality care. These missed opportunities result in unnecessary duplication of errors, harm or substandard health care experiences, as well as unnecessary duplication in the process of developing and trialling improvements.

Economic prosperity

With respect to the health complaints entity, its economic impact is affected by the balance between the direct costs of maintaining itself, the indirect costs of its processes and decisions (for instance, their influence on the cost of health care delivery or workforce availability) and potential savings from reducing the economic burden of preventable adverse events. From an economic perspective, the key advantage of health complaints entities is that they serve as an alternative to extremely costly adversarial legal processes. Health complaints entities can act as a skilled and experienced neutral party, with expertise in resolving issues in a fair, balanced and respectful manner. By minimising the volume of legal proceedings against practitioners and health services, health complaints entities reduce the individual and societal costs associated with medico-legal proceedings (both human and financial). As highlighted earlier in this chapter, in New Zealand such legal action is almost entirely disallowed by law. While such litigation is permissible in Australia, the rate of such action is relatively low by international standards (Anderson et al, 2005; Dauer, 2011).

Within the publicly funded universal health care systems of Australia and New Zealand, it is in the public interest to prevent the direct health care costs, indirect compensation costs and broader economic losses associated with preventable harm in health care. If executed effectively, health complaints entities could play a significant role in achieving this. However, the existence of health complaints entities does come at a financial cost. In particular, matters that proceed to formal investigation can carry a high cost for both the health complaints entity and the parties involved. In order to minimise unnecessary costs, and best serve the economic interests of society, best practice is for health complaints entities to adopt a 'right-touch' approach to complaints handling and regulation.

Professionals, policy makers and regulators of health services in jurisdictions such as Australasia, Canada and the UK are keenly interested in 'right-touch regulation' (College of Registered Nurses of British Columbia, 2012; Bilton and Cayton, 2013; Crocket, 2014; Professional Standards Authority, 2015). According to the UK Professional Standards Authority for Health and Social Care, right-touch regulation is 'based on a proper evaluation of risk, is proportionate and outcome focused; it creates a framework in which professionalism can flourish and organisations can be excellent' (Professional Standards Authority, 2015). Building on the *Principles of Good Regulation* (BRTF, 2003), the Professional Standards Authority developed the following six principles of right-touch regulation:

- *Proportionate:* Regulators should only intervene when necessary. Remedies should be appropriate to the risk posed and costs identified and minimised.
- *Consistent:* Rules and standards must be joined up and implemented fairly.
- *Targeted:* Regulation should be focused on the problem and minimise side-effects.
- *Transparent:* Regulators should be open, and keep regulations simple and user-friendly.
- *Accountable:* Regulators must be able to justify decisions and be subject to public scrutiny.
- *Agile:* Regulation must look forward and be able to adapt and anticipate change.

The right-touch approach aims to ensure that complaints handling and regulation is responsive, adaptive and contextually informed. In particular, it aims to impose regulatory requirements and actions that are as minimally intrusive and restrictive as possible, while still achieving adequate protection for patients. Such an approach to regulation and complaints handling, and thus harm minimisation, is generally an economically efficient one.

Right-touch regulation is 'categorically not "light-touch"'; rather, it aims to strike the right balance by using the minimum regulatory force needed to achieve the desired result' (Professional Standards Authority, 2015: 14). This regulatory approach requires that regulators have at their disposal a range of both lighter, less formal and less punitive actions, as well as more heavy-handed ones. It also requires that they have the discretion, powers and resources to utilise these effectively. Health complaints entities serve a vital role in operating at the 'lighter touch' end of this spectrum, with health workforce regulators and health profession boards occupying the 'heavier-handed' end. When injured patients feel that the entities tasked with resolving their grievances do not meet their needs, they often perceive this as an abdication of public responsibility and describe these entities as 'toothless' or 'paper tigers' (Moore and Mello, 2017). Such sentiments highlight the importance of seeking the right balance between two extremes: under-regulation and over-regulation.

Open justice

The final way in which health complaints entities contribute to the public interest is by enhancing accountability and oversight for health care systems, thus enhancing public trust in those systems. The pursuit of open justice complements and co-exists with the right to a fair trial, and requires that legal proceedings be open to scrutiny by the public and the media. However, open justice may be rightly limited in some situations, for example where it is necessary to protect witnesses, or to maintain confidentiality. Openness in health complaints entities' processes can potentially serve two functions: first, as a window onto the work of the health complaints entity itself; and second, as a 'porthole' through which the public can observe whether the health care system is meeting its obligations to ensure the quality and safety of care.

Overall, public trust in health practitioners in Australia and New Zealand is high, as is support for both countries' public health systems. However, this trust, and trust in health complaints entities, has been challenged by the unsatisfactory experiences of individual patients and complainants, as well as by publicity about high-profile failings of complaints systems to protect patients from harm. In practice, the openness of health complaints entities is limited. Health complaints entities do publish public reports containing data such as the overall number of complaints received, broad themes raised in complaints and complaint resolution timelines. Some reports also include de-identified examples of complaints. However, actionable information such as specific risks, warnings and recommendations are rarely made public. Confidentiality agreements and the legal privilege attached to conciliation also limit openness, restricting the ability of health complaints entities to name and discuss problematic practitioners and services publicly.

Health complaints entities in Australia and New Zealand have also been criticised for a lack of transparency about their processes, including information about their investigative and decision-making processes, as well as processes and communication occurring at the interface between health complaints entities and regulators (Paterson, 2012). For example, there is a lack of transparency regarding the interface between health complaints entities and the practitioner regulation boards, with little information provided to complainants about how or when a complaint might be transferred from one entity to the other. The successful operation of health complaints entities is dependent on public complaints, without which identification of significant risks and issues is difficult. Access to such complaints depends on the public's willingness to make them, which in turn hinges on the public's trust in health complaints entities, and the effectiveness and integrity of their processes and outcomes. Therefore, in order to best serve the public good, it is important that health complaints entities pair the public's trust with matching trustworthiness, and heed the concerns of complainants who are dissatisfied with their experience of health complaints entities' services.

There is great potential value in ensuring that information from health complaints entities, including statistical analyses, case examples, reports of findings, recommendations and warnings, is disseminated widely to both the public and health care providers. One example of how health complaints entities may support open justice, while still protecting the privacy of individual parties, is via the publication of searchable, de-identified case summaries, and associated recommendations, warnings and lessons. This would help to 'close the loop' of information back to health care providers and the health sector at large. It would provide a valuable educational resource for professionals, as well as providing patients with examples of what service standards are acceptable and unacceptable in various circumstances, and how a health complaints entity might assist them.

Challenges and opportunities

In Australia and New Zealand, the work of health complaints entities has improved public awareness about patients' rights, and the availability and importance of complaint mechanisms (Skegg, 2011). Despite these successes, in the previous section we highlighted the challenge presented by the perceived lack of transparency in health complaints entities' processes. In this section, we identify four additional, emerging challenges with important implications and opportunities for the contribution of health complaints entities to the public interest. These are risk-informed practice, data sharing, online health advice and complainant dissatisfaction.

Risk-informed practice

At present, the work of health complaints entities is largely reactive – driven by the complaints that arrive in their offices. Consequently, their work does not often adopt a systematic approach to assessing the risk posed by specific individuals, services or issues, and the relative public harm that may result. Yet research using health complaints entities' data clearly demonstrates that the risk of complaints is unevenly distributed across Australia's medical workforce. A study of over 18,000 complaints to health complaints entities in six of Australia's states and territories found that only 3% of doctors accounted for 49% of complaints (Bismark et al, 2013). The complaint-prone status of these individuals may reflect a heightened risk to patients.

Proactively targeting health complaints entities' resources towards identifying, investigating and addressing the risks posed by such high-risk individuals may result in two key benefits. First, it may improve both the efficiency and effectiveness of health complaints entities by:

- reducing staff workloads (potentially improving the quality of work performed);
- speeding up complaint resolution;
- reducing the time that lower-risk practitioners spend dealing with health complaints entities;
- improving the magnitude of real-world safety improvements resulting from health complaints entities' processes.

Through better risk assessment, it may also reduce the number of cases that health complaints entities refer to regulators, reducing the likelihood of expensive and burdensome regulatory investigations that do not result in regulatory action.

Second, the ability to identify such high-risk individuals using health complaints entities' complaints data provides an opportunity to more proactively protect the public from the potential dangers they pose. However, this opportunity is not well utilised at present. Health complaints entities and staff have expressed frustration and concern that while they are often acutely aware of 'frequent flyers' in their complaints work, they are restricted from issuing specific public statements and warnings about these concerns. In one notable case, then Victorian Health Services Commissioner, Dr Beth Wilson, won a Supreme Court case seeking to publicly name self-professed 'shaman' and 'healer' Peter de Angelis in the Victorian Parliament, on the grounds that he was an ongoing danger to the public. A year-long investigation by the Victorian Health Services Commissioner had revealed a pattern of alleged sexual misconduct against at least six female cancer patients. Following the court's ruling, Dr Wilson named de Angelis in a report to Parliament, exercising powers never previously utilised by her office. Following the de Angelis case, Dr Wilson campaigned for the ability of the Victorian health complaints entity to publicly name offenders earlier, where there are reasonable grounds to believe that they pose a significant and serial risk to the public (Stark, 2012). An expansion of public naming powers is among the powers granted to the new incarnation of Victoria's health complaints entity, which began operation in 2017 as the Health Complaints Commissioner.

Several health complaints entities have shown willingness to engage with researchers to generate evidence to guide their work (Bismark and Studdert, 2010). This direction is promising, and evidence-based complaints management is an important future direction.

Data sharing

One significant obstacle to proactive public protection by health complaints entities and other entities is the fragmentation of complaints and safety data across multiple entities and jurisdictions. For example, multiple complaints or concerns about a practitioner may be spread across employers, health services, regulators, coroners, police, courts, insurers, health complaints entities and other complaints or regulatory agencies (such as consumer rights entities). This can make patterns of concern difficult to detect and act upon. The problem is compounded because records may be spread across multiple states and territories, or even countries.

The ongoing failure to appropriately link and communicate complaints information presents a barrier to early identification and intervention with high-risk practitioners or services. Former gynaecologist Roman Hasil (who practised in both Australia and New Zealand) is an example of this problem (Health and Disability Commissioner, 2008). Across both countries, Hasil was accused of the following: practising while intoxicated and impaired by a head injury, performing procedures without consent, inadequate record-keeping, attempting to practise while not registered, falsifying timesheet entries, and serious medical errors during surgery. The true extent of concerns about Hasil's problematic behaviour, character and competence was long obscured by the many agencies and countries involved. For instance, various agencies held records about Hasil detailing that he was:

- refused registration in Tasmania and South Australia due to criminal records;
- failed by Australian medical examiners three times;
- accused of falsifying timesheet entries by an employer in New South Wales, Australia;
- fired from a hospital in Victoria, Australia for practising while intoxicated;
- the subject of a New Zealand Health and Disability Commissioner inquiry into his work at Whanganui Hospital in 2005-06;
- the subject of complaints about medical negligence and sexual assault at multiple hospitals across Australia and New Zealand.

As a result of the failure of the agencies involved to share this information with each other, and to actively seek out such information, employers and regulators did not 'connect the dots'. Aided by his mobility across states and countries, Hasil continued to cause harm to patients for years, even after serious concerns were raised.

As we move towards a more mobile medical workforce, the ability to access information about practitioners who have previously placed patient safety at risk will become even more important. Improvements in data linkage and information sharing will require improvements in the use of cross-compatible technology, as well as changes in policies, laws, attitudes and institutional and professional culture among a wide range of agencies. If this can be achieved, it will provide an opportunity to not only detect patterns of concern, but also to empower health complaints entities to access information that can confirm or refute the claims made by complainants and respondents during complaints processes. For example, complaints regarding prescribing behaviour will be more easily informed by immediate and direct access to information from national prescribing and medication services, such as Australia's Pharmaceutical Benefits Scheme.

Online health advice

Health complaints entities can receive complaints about widely recognised professions that are not covered by regulators (such as social workers, counsellors and speech pathologists), as well as individuals who offer health services under less-recognised titles (such as 'faith healer' or 'shaman'), or no specific title at all. An emerging challenge for health complaints entities in protecting the public stems from the increasing prevalence and impact of health advice provided online by individuals who are not registered health practitioners, such as 'health bloggers'. It is unclear if and when such advice constitutes a 'health service' as defined by the policies and legislation governing the scope of health complaints entities. These individuals can wield influence over the health behaviours of many individuals and receive payment or other financial benefits for doing so. An example of such an individual is former Australian health blogger Belle Gibson, who has been subject to court action by the consumers' rights organisation Consumer Affairs Victoria, following allegations of fraud in the operation of her blog, app, book and charity (Donelly and Toscano, 2016). The potential role for health complaints entities in managing complaints about similar incidents is unclear, but will likely be tested in the future.

Complainant dissatisfaction

As discussed in the earlier section on health complaints entities and the public interest, the potential benefits for individual complainants are not currently being fully realised. Surveys have shown that many individual patients interacting with health complaints entities are dissatisfied with their experience (Daniel et al, 1999). One important explanation for this dissatisfaction is an 'expectations gap' (Bismark et al, 2011; Dauer, 2011) – that is, discord between what complainants want and what they eventually get out of the process. A published analysis of 189 complaints to the Office of the Health Services Commissioner in Victoria, Australia, provided evidence of such a gap (Bismark et al, 2011). Among the complainants, only a third who sought restoration received it and only one in five who sought correction received assurances that changes had been or would be made to reduce the risk of others experiencing similar harm. Finally, less than one in ten who sought sanctions saw at least the initial steps taken to achieve this outcome. It was concluded that bridging this expectations gap may help to improve complainant satisfaction with complaints systems.

There remain questions about the appropriateness of complainant satisfaction as a metric for evaluating the success of health complaints entities. According to Weisfeld, an American commentator, the 'ultimate test' of complaints mechanisms is 'whether they help lead to an improved healthcare system, not whether they satisfy established constituencies in the short run' (Paterson, 2002: 73). Our view is that these goals are inextricably connected. Given that health complaints entities are patient-centred, and an important statutory purpose of these entities is the protection and promotion of patients' rights, it is vital to include patients' views in evaluations of health complaints entities. Such patient involvement may contribute towards improved health complaints entities and the overall health care system. The ongoing challenge lies in ensuring that patients are conceptualised as partners (rather than adversaries), who may work with practitioners and entities to achieve these goals.

Conclusion

The dominant discourse regarding medical regulation often presents the interests of health providers in competition with the opposing interests of patients and the public. The assumption is that one 'side' will always lose out in regulatory decision making and policy development. However, Australia and New Zealand's experience with health complaints entities demonstrates that practitioners, patients and the public all stand to gain from fair, timely and cost-effective complaint resolution processes that address the needs of individual patients, while also disseminating the lessons learned and identifying problematic practitioners. Professional cultures that encourage open engagement with health complaints entities are vital to overcoming the barriers posed by the often voluntary nature of their processes. Appropriate complaint resolution and service improvement can result when practitioners and services have effective complaints-handling mechanisms, as well as receptive, constructive attitudes towards complaints. The unfinished business lies in realising the full potential of health complaints entities to serve the public's interest in enhancing transparency and accountability, as well as patient safety.

Notes

1. In this chapter, we use the term 'health complaints entities', rather than 'health complaints commissions', because 'health complaints entity' is the terminology used in the Australian National Scheme. We use 'commissioner(s)' when referring to a specific health complaints entity such as the New Zealand Health and Disability Commissioner.

2. In this chapter, we use the term 'patients' to broadly cover patients as well as their relatives, friends and carers. In keeping with the New Zealand statutory language, we also recognise that the terms 'consumers' or 'clients' may be more appropriate than 'patients' in some contexts.

Acknowledgements

The authors are grateful to Professor Ron Paterson and the editors of this volume for their insightful comments on earlier drafts of this chapter.

References

Anderson, G., Hussey, P., Frognerm, B. and Waters, H. (2005) 'Health spending in the United States and the rest of the industrialised world', *Health Affairs* 24: 903-14.

Australian Commission on Safety and Quality in Healthcare (2008) 'Australian Charter of Healthcare Rights', https://www.safetyandquality.gov.au/national-priorities/charter-of-healthcare-rights/

Australian Law Reform Commission (2014) *Serious Invasions of Privacy in the Digital Era: Discussion Paper 80 (DP 80)*, Sydney: Australian Law Reform Commission .

Beaupert, F., Carney, T., Chiarella, M., Satchell, C., Walton, M., Bennett, B. and Kelly, P. (2014) 'Regulating health care complaints: a literature review', *International Journal of Health Care Quality Assurance* 27: 505-18.

Bilton, D. and Cayton, H. (2013) 'Finding the right touch: extending the right-touch regulation approach to the accreditation of voluntary registers', *British Journal of Guidance and Counselling* 41(1): 14-23.

Bismark, M., Spittal, M., Gogos, A., Gruen, R. and Studdert, D. (2011) 'Remedies sought and obtained in healthcare complaints', *BMJ Quality and Safety* 20: 806-10.

Bismark, M., Spittal, M., Gurrin, L., Ward, M. and Studdert, D. (2013) 'Identification of doctors at risk of recurrent complaints: a national study of healthcare complaints in Australia', *BMJ Quality and Safety* 22: 532-40.

Bismark, M. and Studdert, D. (2010) 'Realising the research power of complaints data', *New Zealand Medical Journal* 123(1314): 12-17.

Brennan, T., Leape, L., Laird, N., Hebert, L., Localio, A., Lawthers, A., Newhouse, J., Weiler, P. and Hiatt, H. (1991) 'Incidence of adverse events and negligence in hospitalized patients: results of the Harvard medical practice study I', *New England Journal of Medicine* 324: 370-6.

BRTF (Better Regulation Task Force) (2003) *Principles of Good Regulation*, London: BRTF.

Cartwright, S. (1988) *The Report of the Cervical Cancer Inquiry*, Auckland, New Zealand: Government Printing Office.

Chamberlain, J. M. (2013) *The Sociology of Medical Regulation: An Introduction*, London: Springer.

College of Registered Nurses of British Columbia (2012) *Underlying Philosophies and Trends Affecting Professional Regulation*, British Columbia, Canada: College of Registered Nurses of British Columbia.

Crocket, A. (2014) 'Recognition, regulation, registration: seeking the right touch', *New Zealand Journal of Counselling* 34(1): 53-68.

Daniel, A., Burn, R. and Horarik, S. (1999) 'Patients' complaints about medical practice', *Medical Journal of Australia* 170: 598-602.

Dauer, E. (2011) 'Medical injury, patients' claims and the effects of government responses in Anglo–American legal systems', *BMJ Quality and Safety* 20: 735-7.

Dew, K. and Roorda, M. (2001) 'Institutional innovation and the handling of health complaints in New Zealand: an assessment', *Health Policy* 57: 27-44.

Donelly, B. and Toscano, N. (2016) 'Conwoman Belle Gibson faces $1m fines over cancer scam fundraising fraud', *The Age* 6 May, https://www.theage.com.au/national/victoria/cancer-conwoman-belle-gibson-faces-1m-fines-over-fundraising-scam-20160428-goh3r2.html

Fallberg, L. and MacKenney, S. (2003) 'Patient ombudsmen in seven European countries: an effective way to implement patients' rights?', *European Journal of Health Law* 10: 343-57.

HDC (Health and Disability Commissioner) (2008) *Dr Roman Hasil and Whanganui District Health Board 2005-2006*, Auckland, New Zealand: HDC.

HDC (2014) *Health and Disability Commissioner Annual Report*, Auckland, New Zealand: HDC.

HDC (2016) *The Health and Disability Commissioner – The HDC Code of Health and Disability Services Consumers' Rights Regulation 1996*, Auckland, New Zealand: HDC, www.hdc.org.nz/the-act--code

Madden, B. (2016) 'The national disability insurance scheme: advice on compensation recovery', *Law Society of New South Wales Journal* 29: 90-1.

Moore, J. and Mello, M. M. (2017) 'Improving reconciliation following medical injury: a qualitative study of responses to patient safety incidents in New Zealand', *BMJ Quality and Safety*, 10.1136/bmjqs-2016-005804

Moore, J., Bismark, M. and Mello, M. M. (2017) 'Patients' experiences with communication-and-resolution programs after medical injury', *JAMA Internal Medicine* 177(11): 1595-1603.

Nettleton, S. and Harding, G. (1994) 'Protesting patients: a study of complaints submitted to a family health service authority', *Sociology of Health and Illness* 16: 38-61.

Paterson, R. (2002) 'The patients' complaints system in New Zealand', *Health Affairs* 21: 70-9.

Paterson, R. (2008) 'Inquiries into health care: learning or lynching?', *New Zealand Medical Journal* 121: 100-15.

Paterson, R. (2012) *The Good Doctor: What Patients Want*, Auckland, New Zealand: Auckland University Press.

Paterson, R. (2015) 'Complaints, investigations and compensation', in Skegg, P. and Paterson, R. (eds) *Health Law in New Zealand*, Wellington, New Zealand: Thomson Reuters.

Paterson, R. and Manning, J. (2017) 'Complaint resolution, quality improvement and public protection: the diverse roles of Australasian health complaints entities', in Freckelton, I. and Petersen, K. (eds) *Tensions and Traumas in Health Law*, Sydney, Australia: Federation Press.

Professional Standards Authority (2015) *Right-Touch Regulation: Revised*, London: PSA.

Rosenthal, M. (1992) 'Medical discipline in cross-cultural perspective: the United States, Britain and Sweden', in Dingwall, R. and Fenn, P. (eds) *Quality and Regulation in Health Care*, London: Routledge.

Skegg, P. (2011) 'A fortunate experiment? New Zealand's experience with a legislated code of patients' rights', *Medical Law Review* 19: 235-66.

Stark, J. (2012) 'The right medicine', *The Age* 20 May, https://www.theage.com.au/national/victoria/the-right-medicine-20120519-1yxpv.html

Wall, J. (2016) 'In what sense "rights"? Principles of justice and the Code of Patients' Rights', in Henaghan, M. and Wall, J. (eds) *Law, Ethics and Medicine: Essays in Honour of Peter Skegg*, Wellington, New Zealand: Thomson Reuters.

THIRTEEN

Trust and the regulation of health systems: insights from India

Michael Calnan and Sumit Kane

Introduction

At the heart of the regulatory enterprise is the intention to control the behaviour of actors to achieve a variety of economic objectives and social objectives in the public interest. This chapter examines the current regulatory regimes and practices in the health system in India, using the trust/control duality as an analytical frame. In doing so, it critically reflects on the stewardship and governance of the health system, exposing the limits and fragilities of the current regulatory approach to controlling health system actors' behaviours and practices. Evidence and insights from this analysis are used to depict the nature of trust relations and regulation in the health system, and the problems therein, and to explain why they take that shape. The final part of the chapter outlines possible strategies for the effective stewardship and governance of health systems, and concludes with the identification of key questions for further research.

Rationales for regulation

Regulation as an intervention is usually the prerogative of governments. While politically, governments may have many possible motives behind regulating or not, on a purely technical level, the rationale behind regulation as an intervention is the pursuit of the public interest. Two broad rationales are identified for regulation in the health care context. The first major rationale is that health care markets are imperfect markets and are prone to a range of market failures that require control and intervention to protect the public interest; and also that the health care market is an imperfect market with many public goods, merit goods and private goods with positive and negative externalities,[1] all requiring some form of intervention to promote the public interest.

The second major rationale locates regulation prior to, and not in response to, market failures. In this rationale, regulation is seen as a method for organising social relations as a matter of right and as an expression of and a means to furthering social solidarity.

The market failure and imperfect markets rationale for regulation addresses certain unique properties of the health care market. For example, in the health care market, the providers are from professions where entry is very restrictive; this restricted entry to the supply side of the health care market very often creates situations of monopolies or oligopolies with little or no room for competition; this structurally places limitations on options that patients, organisations and populations might have in terms of the choice of providers in a particular context – requiring intervention to protect the public interest. Similarly, in a well-functioning competitive market, consumers are well informed, can evaluate competing products and can make informed decisions about their own needs and requirements. However, it has been argued that ill-health and health care are distinctively characterised by unpredictability and uncertainty, and so are not easily commodified (Titmuss, 2004). Thus, in the health care market, it is almost always the provider who, mainly by virtue of access to specialist knowledge, defines and decides the needs of the consumer-patient. This information asymmetry and unequal bargaining and negotiating power requires intervention to protect the public interest from what is called 'provider-side moral hazard'.

The rights and social solidarity rationale for regulation addresses social concerns related to distributional justice, the protection of rights and the prevention of discrimination based on race, gender or age, and is located within the broader social and citizenship compact of a particular society. For instance, intervention in the form of regulation is often required to ensure the accessibility of health and other facilities for people with physical disabilities; similarly in some contexts, interventions are instituted to control the pricing of services either generally or for specific diseases or population groups.

Some of the market failure rationales and the social solidarity/greater good rationales for regulatory intervention also overlap. For instance, markets work best when the price of a product or a service encompasses all of the benefits of the particular product. However, in the health care market there are many treatments, for example the treatment of infectious diseases, which benefit not just the individual, but also wider populations, and vice versa. These externalities, both positive and negative, serve as a rationale for intervention. Similarly, in the health care market there are goods that if left to the devices of market forces, are unlikely to be purchased and consumed by people, but are such that for the greater societal good, should be consumed; so the promotion of the consumption of these merit goods requires intervention. For example, if people were asked to pay for the multiple rounds of polio vaccines that are needed to achieve herd immunity for global polio elimination, they would likely not if their child had been vaccinated already; intervention is required either to insist on vaccination or to make the services free, or as is often the case, both.

Regulation of the health sector in India

India has a pluralistic health system made up of a mix of public, private for-profit and private not-for-profit financers and providers. People living in poverty use primary care services in both the public and the private sectors, while more affluent people use these only in the private sector. However, more affluent people also use specialist services provided by the public sector, and people living in poverty can only access these services in the public sector (Minocha, 1980; de Costa et al, 2008). The Indian health system is characterised by a multitude of regulations introduced on the basis of both of the rationales discussed in the previous section. They have been incrementally introduced over the past few decades, as policies and regulations tend to be in democratic societies, in response to events, disasters and failures, and the public discourses around these. While it is beyond the scope of this chapter to provide a detailed account, this section briefly describes the complex health care regulatory environment in India.

Broadly, separate sets of regulations target professionals and health care facilities in the public and private sectors, the wider profession and the pharmaceuticals market. The National Health Bill 2009 serves as the instrument for the regulation of public health services and is implemented through the national and state health boards. These boards regulate various aspects of service provision and research through the development of practice standards, protocols, norms and guidelines.

While the National Health Bill 2009 also includes some regulatory oversight of the private sector, the Clinical Establishments (Registration and Regulation) Act 2010 and the Bombay Public Trust Act 1950 are major instruments for the regulation of the private health sector. In parallel, the Quality Council of India, a non-statutory body, through its National Accreditation Board for Hospitals and Healthcare Providers (NABH) also develops standards for hospitals and health care providers. NABH accredits health care services; NABH accreditation is voluntary and can be sought by public and private providers. Another major regulation governing the private health care sector in India is the Consumer Protection Act 1986. This redefines the provider–patient relationship as a provider–consumer relationship and puts in place measures for the protection of the rights of consumers of health care providers' services. While these regulations tend to have a broad remit, there are many regulations that target specific aspects of health care provision. For example, the Pre-Conception and Pre-Natal Diagnostic Technique Act (PC and PNDT) 1994 regulates ultrasonography services with a view to preventing the detection of the foetus's sex in order to check female foeticide. Similarly, the Medical Termination of Pregnancy Act 1971 regulates the provision of abortion services.

In addition to all of the above, the medical profession is regulated via the Medical Council of India (MCI) Act 1956. The MCI Act has provisions and specific regulations for professional standards, conduct standards, training and practice standards, registration and ethical standards. Similarly, the pharmaceutical industry is regulated by a number of regulations from across industry, drugs, food and medicine domains. The federal nature of India's polity adds to the complexity of the regulatory environment of the health sector; both the central and state legislatures can legislate on most matters related to 'health'. Many regulations promulgated at the centre may not be effected by the states, or may be effected partially/differently.

Regulatory failures

The complex regulatory environment notwithstanding, given that regulations are primarily interventions to control the behaviours and practices of actors, they tend to be prone to failure. Regulations can fail due to many reasons. They can:

- fail to *detect* undesirable and noncompliant practices;
- fail to *respond* by developing appropriate policies, rules and tools to deal with the problems discovered;
- fail to *enforce* the policies, rules and tools on the ground;
- fail to *assess* and measure success or failure in enforcement activities;
- fail to *modify* tools and strategies in order to improve compliance and address problematic practice.
  (Baldwin and Black, 2008)

Furthermore, regulations are also prone to being captured by interest groups and the selective application of regulations due, for example, to bureaucratic self-interest, thereby undermining the original purpose of the regulation.

Researchers from India (for instance, Bloom et al, 2008; Peters and Muraleedharan, 2008; Kane and Calnan, 2016) have shown that many of the regulations in the Indian health system are well intentioned, yet they continue to fail to achieve their goals. These researchers have also pointed out that these failures occur at multiple levels, ranging from systemic and design failures to implementation failures. Peters and Muraleedharan (2008) argue that the highly control-oriented 'inspectorate raj' nature of the regulatory model, focused on enforcing rules, makes the regulatory model in India particularly vulnerable to failure. Different types of regulatory failures experienced in the Indian health system are illustrated through the following examples from different health policy and practice domains.

Regulatory failures in the Indian health system: some examples

Examples are drawn from three domains:

- the privatisation of medical education;
- for-profit private provision of health services;
- failures in implementing and enforcing existing regulations.

For each of the three domains, a brief overview is initially presented of the state of affairs, drawing on the existing literature to highlight failures, primarily at the policy level. This is followed by reflections on this, mainly at the policy and practice implementation level, based on insights from data[2] from a recent study about trust in health care in India, specifically drawing on interviews with medical doctors, health care managers, civil society actors, local politicians and citizens (Kane et al, 2015). These examples from the health policy and practice domains highlight the complexity of the issues, actors and perspectives involved in the process of regulating the health system in India.

The case of the privatisation of medical education

To address the chronic and critical shortages in human resources for health, within the ambit of existing regulatory frameworks, policies were introduced to allow the private sector to provide medical education in India. Today more than 50% of the medical schools in India are privately owned or managed. Over the past two decades, problems have been highlighted by both the mainstream media and academia (Arora, 2016; Phadke, 2016) about how the existing regulations related to medical education in India are not complied with, are insufficient, and prone to capture and abuse by interest groups. Dramatic cases of poor-quality education, non-compliance with standards and the outright sale of undergraduate and postgraduate places, have been regularly reported. In spite of this increasing awareness, as Phadke (2016) argues, the current regulatory regime continues to fail to be effective both because of its inability to sufficiently modify strategies to improve compliance and address problematic practices, and due perhaps to the inappropriateness of the policies, rules and tools to deal with the problems discovered.

This is exemplified by informants in the study who felt strongly about the current situation. Their view was that the proliferation of for-profit private medical colleges, and the poor oversight of these, was central to understanding the current state of the profession. These informants pointed out how people in society were well aware that gaining admissions into these medical colleges was not about fulfilling academic criteria and merit, but rather about having the resources to bribe and buy the admissions process: "Ever since these private colleges have opened, there is an element of doubt. People obviously have doubts … [they wonder] if this doctor has actually seen any patients at all" (Civil Society Informant).

According to these informants, such practices, and the impunity with which the regulations governing admissions to medical colleges were ignored and circumvented by the affluent and powerful, have created doubts in people's minds about the competence of doctors, their intentions given the vast bribes involved, and the stewardship of the health system:

> '[There are] … those who are coming new. Those who don't deserve admission in the medical colleges and they get admission by hook or crook. People now wonder … where did you study? … people wonder if this doctor is someone who got admitted into medical training just paying money … they wonder if he is someone who paid for his grades … whether he has really studied anything at all.' (Private provider)

The case of the for-profit private provision of health services

During the 1980s, it became recognised that access to health care for the population as a whole was constrained to a large extent by the undersupply of health services. In view of the inability of the state to address this problem of undersupply, in 1986, the hospital sector was declared an industry and a variety of privileges and incentives were provided for private players to become actively involved in all aspects and levels of health care provision (Baru, 2006). The state, however, failed to anticipate the complexity of this development, and as the private sector grew, so did the problems associated with it. These problems included but were not limited to:

- overcharging for services;
- price fixing;
- giving and receiving bribes for referrals;
- favours and bribes from pharmaceutical companies (D'Cruz and Bharat, 2001; Bloom et al, 2008; Sen and Iyer, 2015; Phadke, 2016).

While it has taken years for regulatory responses and tools to be developed, most of these problems remain unaddressed. In addition, whichever regulatory responses have been instituted, their implementation is insufficiently resourced; this has tended to undermine their effectiveness. Furthermore, there are increasing reports (Arora, 2016; Phadke, 2016) of a lack of assessment of the success or failure of the enforcement activities of regulators; this is particularly problematic in light of street-level bureaucrats selectively applying regulations to enhance their self-interest, thereby further undermining the original intentions and goals of the regulations.

Among the informants in the study, both the civil society representative and the politician categorically stated that people were well aware of the various malpractices prevalent in the medical profession. The following quotations from their interviews highlight that a social discourse, wherein people distrust the intentions of large sections of the medical profession and simultaneously distrust the competence of the regulatory apparatus to check this moral hazard, is gaining ground.

> 'There is definitely a certain element of doubt, particularly in urban areas. There is talk of irrational practices, unnecessary investigations, unnecessary surgeries [all to make money] ... how the private sector is exploitative. There are lots of articles in newspapers too ... because of that, a discourse [f distrust of the profession and ineffectiveness of the regulatory apparatus] has taken root.' (Civil society)

> 'Doctors have their eyes set on what they can get [from the pharmaceutical companies] ... the [international] conferences they can travel to. Yes, the pharmaceutical companies pay; the doctors prescribe [their] medicines, and the pharmaceutical companies pay for these expenses. People in society know [about this nexus], perhaps not those who are illiterate, but people know.' (Politician)

However, unlike the civil society representative and the politician, as illustrated by the quotation below and discussed in detail elsewhere (Kane et al, 2015), some citizen informants appeared to be far less critical of the medical profession and its regulation. They seemed confident that *their* doctors would safeguard their interests, in spite of being aware of the unethical practices. This paradox could be explained at multiple levels:

- it could reflect the low expectations that these particular informants had from those mandated with the stewardship role and for guarding their interests;
- it could reflect a sense of resigned acceptance of the ineffectiveness of the regulators;
- it could also indicate the priorities that people accord to different aspects of the provider–patient relationship, and the tacit understandings they might have with their doctors about the trade-offs they are willing to make and accept given the circumstances.

> 'Not really ... I don't feel that way because ... they must have their own problems, that is why they take ... a little bit is OK. After all it is someone's occupation ... as a doctor [occupation] they have got to make money.' (Citizen)

The case of failures in implementing and enforcing existing regulations

The distrust engendered by the above failures is further amplified by the way authorities address the interpretation and implementation of the regulations. The recent nationwide strike (*Indian Express*, 2016) by radiologists against the way the Pre-Conception and Pre-Natal Diagnostic Technique (PC and PNDT) Act 1994 is being implemented, and the recently launched petition by the Indian Medical Association against what it calls the 'black laws' and 'deceit' of the current regulatory regime (Indian Medical Association, 2016), illustrate both the discontent among the medical professionals with the current state of affairs and the gravity of the situation. The strongest critics of the Indian Medical Association's resistance to any attempts at regulation of the profession (Phadke, 2010; Phadke, 2016), suggest that the Association 'has morphed into a body representing the trade and commerce of medicine rather than the practice of medicine as a whole' (Nagral, 2012), but also recognise the problems with the way the authorities have interpreted and sought to enforce the various regulations, particularly the Clinical Establishment Act 2010 and the PC and PNDT Act. That radiologists in India have had to resort to nationwide industrial action, and that the association of radiologists had support from both the Federation of Obstetrics and Gynaecology Society of India and the Indian Medical Association, signals a state of deep distrust between the medical professionals and the regulators. This state of affairs, Nagral's contention notwithstanding, is also the product of regulatory failures, and clearly appears unproductive for all, including for patients.

This state of almost a complete breakdown of trust between providers and regulators was a dominant theme in the study by Kane et al (2015). The following quotation from one of the informants, an obstetrician, about the conduct of the officers involved in implementing the Clinical Establishment Act and the PC and PNDT Act, sums up what is considered a widely held view among the private health care providers in India, including all those interviewed:

> 'If there is someone [some doctor] who is trying to walk the straight path ... they [regulators] will give him all the trouble. [They will] create hurdles at every step. This is how it is ... and the only reason behind it is filling their own pockets.... There is nothing else to it.' (Private provider – obstetrician)

Another informant, a doctor and health services manager, added that the feeling of distrust was mutual; that it was as much driven by perception, as by experience. He contended that, on the one hand, private providers consider every officer involved in the regulatory process to be corrupt, and, on the other hand, most officers also approach private providers with a view that they are involved in malpractices:

> 'The first assumption is that they are not following the rules and regulations and therefore it is always suspicious. [There

is] suspicion on both side. [There is] distrust, the perception
… it starts with distrust. And here in private practice …
[doctors] distrust every officer … every regulator is corrupt.'
(Health services manager – medical doctor)

A further example, of regulatory approaches and practices being captured by interest groups and the failure of the state to detect and respond to this in an appropriate and timely manner, is the case of the failure of the professional bodies mandated with the self-regulation of the medical profession. The Medical Council of India has over the past two decades been embroiled in a series of scandals, all centred around its failure to uphold its mandate and abuse of entrusted power (Chatterjee, 2010; Sachan, 2013; Vijaykumar and Saini, 2013; Tiwari, 2015). Not only has the response been slow, it might also be argued that it has been consistently unimaginative, if not inappropriate, each time responding with ever-greater control measures and with ever-greater force (Sen and Iyer, 2015). In the most recent iteration, in 2016, in a dramatic turn of events, a recent report of the Parliamentary Standing Committee on Health and Family Welfare on the functioning of the MCI, criticised it for corruption, incompetence and the dereliction of duties, and noted that 'the Medical Council of India … has repeatedly failed on all its mandates over the decades', and that the state of the medical profession is perhaps at its 'lowest ebb' (Rajya Sabha, 2016: 15). The Supreme Court of India also intervened using its rare and extraordinary powers under the Constitution, to set up a three-member committee headed by a former Chief Justice of India, to oversee the process of overhauling the regulatory framework of the medical profession (Sikri, 2016). This, given the past experience, and given the mandate and make-up of the committee, is likely to be another attempt at exercising ever-greater control.

Remedying regulatory failures: the need to rebuild trust?

Typical remedial approaches to regulatory failures tend to be centred around improving coordination among actors, organisational learning and reform, and modifications to existing regulatory arrangements. Remedial action is important as, whether occurring by deliberate action or by inaction, regulatory failures undermine trust and confidence in governments and institutions mandated with the regulatory function. It is argued here that regulatory failures are in many ways, at a fundamental level, failures of trust and that remedial action for regulatory failures requires the focus to be beyond merely proposing better and more effective ways for exerting greater control, but rather to also frame some of these failures as failures of trust with policy and social responses directed towards rebuilding organisational and institutional trust. This argument is consistent with the large and growing body of theoretical and empirical work examining the trust/control duality, and strategies aimed at repairing trust at the organisational and institutional trust levels.

Cultures of trust and the link with modes of governance

Analysis at the theoretical level has suggested that cultures of trust are associated with different forms of governance (Brown and Calnan, 2016b). For example, Calnan and Rowe (2008), in their typology of governance, identified five different types: market, New Public Management, bureaucratic, professional and stakeholder. They analyse these different types of governance in terms of two different dimensions: levels of public trust and the extent of state control. The market approach, with its emphasis on exchange relations, choice and incentives, is associated with low state control through dispersed consumer control and low levels of trust. Similarly, the public management approach is associated with low levels of trust, but more centralised managerial control where performances needs to be explicitly accounted for. The other three types of governance are associated with higher levels of trust, but varying degrees of state control. The command and control form of governance associated with the bureaucratic model is linked with high levels of trust based on trust in public service values and ethos and professionalism. The other two types are associated with low state control with the professional type, with its emphasis on network relations based on trust and mutual reciprocity, leaving the medical profession to self-regulate as there is high trust in professional norms and expertise. This dispersed – as opposed to centralised – power is also associated with the stakeholder type of governance where there is trust in partners' respect of reciprocal rights and duties, but in this context the need for accountability is made explicit, which stands in contrast to the professional type of governance where accountability is implicit.

Clearly, to repair trust then requires an approach to governance that enhances a culture of trust, which suggests that the preferred type might be a form of stakeholder governance where there is mutual trust, but with an emphasis on explicit accountability and transparency. The question is whether it suits the socio-political and cultural context of the health system in India. Certainly, the role of governance may now be changing with the rise of corporate organisations, with a movement away from small medical practices, and the emergence of health insurance companies as important purchasers of care. These changes may necessitate different governance regimes, with increasing emphasis on partnership between the state, market players and civil society organisations involving the so-called co–production of regulatory arrangements (Bloom et al, 2008).

It is also important to distinguish between different levels or layers of trust at the macro, meso and micro levels, which might be termed institutional, organisational and interpersonal trust relations. Much of the argument in this chapter so far has tended to focus at the institutional level, with a particular emphasis on governance and cultures of trust. This institutional level of trust is referred to by some authors (Pilgrim et al, 2010: 9) as systems trust, which relates to 'accountability and the checks and balances and systems that maintain fairness, preventing incompetence or malign intent'. This primarily involves the relationships between the regulators and the professional associations and practitioners who provide the service. Thus, it is argued that: 'Trust, in its different dimensions, is essential to functioning relationships at different levels of health systems through establishing shared norms and values, reputation and legitimacy' (Bloom et al, 2008: 2085). However, organisational and patient–clinician trust relations are also salient in this context. Organisational trust tends to refer to the trust relations between the organisational workforce and, in the context of health care, particularly the relationships between managers and clinicians. It has been argued that in the organisational perspective, trust is important in its own right – that is, it is intrinsically important for the provision of effective health care and has even been described as a collective good, like social trust or social capital (Khodyakov, 2007). Specific organisational benefits that might be derived from trust as a form of social capital include the reduction in transaction costs due to lower surveillance and monitoring costs and the general enhancement of efficiency. In addition, with the increasing use of shared care for patient management, trust between clinicians is even more important, with reliability as well as honesty and competence having been shown to be important components of trust (Calnan and Rowe, 2008).

Trust relations at the micro level between clinicians and patients have been shown to be particularly important for both parties, not least because levels of patient trust have been shown to be both a marker of patients' assessment of the quality of care and related to consultation behaviour, disclosure of information and adherence to medication regimes – and may have a longer-term impact on health outcomes either indirectly or directly through the therapeutic effects of the quality of the trusting relationship (Calnan and Rowe, 2008; Douglass and Calnan, 2016). Public trust in health systems appears to include experiences and perceptions of clinicians as they may be seen to be doing the face work for the health services at the local level, but may also be broader than relationships between patients and providers to include health care systems and socio-political systems that shape cultural beliefs and values about health and health care. These in turn may be influenced by the agenda setting of the media and framing activities in relation to the portrayal of the images of health and health care.

These different levels of layers of trust should not be seen in isolation as there is increasing evidence that they are interrelated and problems at one level may have a knock-on effect at another level. Concentrating primarily on organisational trust, Gilson and colleagues (2005) put forward a conceptual framework that suggests that relations and levels of trust are interconnected. The authors argue that workplace trust shapes the attitudes and practices of health care workers towards patients, which subsequently shapes patient (dis)trust in health care workers. Workplace trust is rooted in micro- and macro-level trust relations, including trust in the employing organisation, trust in one's supervisor and trust in colleagues. Patient trust in health care workers is grounded in interpersonal trust, including the beliefs and behaviour but also the characteristics of the health care worker. The strength of these relations can directly influence patients' trust in providers by shaping their perceptions of the technical competence and fairness of the providers. Providers may end up, due to system and organisational pressures, adopting uncaring attitudes towards patients, which can quickly get entrenched through the formalisation of practices such as defensive treatments and investigations, and unnecessarily involving other specialists. Patient trust may also reflect institutional or system trust, which is rooted in various elements that ensure that health care workers are able to provide care (for example, qualifications and professional codes). Some of these elements may be taken for granted in a context where this level of trust, such as public trust in institutions, is not problematised.

In another example, Brown and Calnan (2016a) also argue that relations and levels of trust are interconnected, in what they call chains of (dis)trust, which provide an explanatory link between trust relations at the organisational level with the quality of patient care. The authors attempt to specify the processes and procedures that account for the nature and structure of these so-called chains of trust relations. Their empirical work was carried out in the clinical setting of the management and treatment of people diagnosed with psychotic mental health problems where there is considerable uncertainty and vulnerability, and thus trust relations tend to be fragile and contested. This research shows how relational-communicative and instrumental-strategic approaches shape the extent to which trust chains could be characterised in terms of a vicious spiral of distrust, or a virtuous cycle of trust. The authors suggest that the conceptual tool of 'trust chains' should not only be characterised as 'link by link' through interpersonal relations, but that in some contexts, institutional and policy directives have shaped trust relations between managers and professionals, even when there was little direct social interaction. It should also be emphasised that such chains in trust relationships may not be necessarily linear nor top down but negotiated where patients play a more active role in shaping the nature of trust relations (Douglass and Calnan, 2016).

The literature, thus, suggests that problems or failures at the institutional and organisational level, leading to a breakdown in trust relations in the health workforce, may influence the quality of patient–provider relationships and levels of trust in those relationships (Gilson et al, 2005).

The trust/control duality

It is evident from the previous section that more directive regulatory interventions such as command and control associated with the New Public Management, and/or marketisation, are not necessarily associated with a culture of high trust. For example, the command and control approach, with its emphasis on performance management, or the incentivising control approach, with its emphasis on choice and competition, adopted in the early part of the century in the English NHS, had limited success, not least because they appeared to have an adverse impact on trust (Brown and Calnan, 2010, 2011). These approaches have tended to focus on the element of trust associated with confidence (associated with competence in carrying out the work), but neglected the relational aspects associated with trust.

This leads on to the more fundamental nature of trust and what type of trust relations policies might be pursued. The previous paragraph highlighted the difference between competence and intentional trust and the evidence suggests that the former tends to form part of or is embedded in the latter – that is, competence makes up an element of more generalised trust (Calnan and Rowe, 2008). However, the previous section depicting the possible relationship between governance and cultures of trust portrayed regulatory approaches, which were associated with higher cultures of trust. There are considerable benefits, as has been outlined earlier, of high trust cultures, but there are also drawbacks. For example, Calnan and Rowe (2008) point to the dark side of trust and a number of different possible costs and dangers associated with it. One of the most relevant in this context is that high trust cultures, possibly associated with self-regulation, may offer the opportunity to exploit the lack of vigilance and assessment and cosy relationships may inhibit innovation and encourage corrupt practices. Thus, it is important to take into account the costs and benefits of trusting relationships and developing an approach to trust that facilitates positive health care performance, but deters exploitation and the abuse of power. Hence, recent commentators have highlighted the importance of the need to develop policies that encourage learnt, informed or critical trust as opposed to blind or assumed trust. There is thus the need for a balance between control and trust, where the latter may encourage reliance and not dependence (Calnan and Rowe, 2008).

Approaches to addressing regulatory failures: repairing trust in organisations and institutions

In view of the arguments in the above sections, the current responses to the many regulatory failures require some reflection and evaluation. It is argued that one should approach with caution policy responses that seek greater control and more regulation alone and that perhaps some of the regulatory failures need to be tackled differently with approaches that entail rebuilding and maintaining trust. For example, as Mollering (2001) argues, a control-based approach works only when the person's positive expectations are based solely on structural influences as the basis for either benevolent or malevolent action. However, when a person's positive expectations are also based on an assumption of benevolent agency or altruistic motives on the part of the other, a trust-based approach, and not a control-based approach, is more appropriate. The latter requires and entails approaches that encourage earned, informed or critical trust.

Continuing with the case of the medical profession in India, the current policy response to the many regulatory failures is to institute greater and stronger regulations. Elsewhere we have argued that policy responses need to focus both on strengthening regulation and on rebuilding trust through interventions that promote conditional and earned trust, while at the same time ensuring that the altruistic intentions and patient-centred orientation of doctors are not undermined (Kane and Calnan, 2016). While the current state of evidence on interventions to improve trust in doctors and in health services is inconclusive (Rolfe et al, 2006), insights from organisational studies (Bachman et al, 2015) provide useful guidance on approaches to repairing and maintaining trust in institutions, including but not limited to those mandated with the stewardship of the health system (for example, regulatory bodies). Bachman and colleagues (2015) propose a model wherein a combination of one or more of six key approaches is deemed necessary to repair, rebuild and maintain trust in institutions in society. These approaches, summarised in Table 13.1, are not all at the same level; they also include regulation and control as an option aimed at external stakeholders, with others aimed at more relational elements.

Table 13.1: Approaches for restoring institutional trust

Sense making	Entails unpacking the reasons for failures and understanding what needs to be done to improve and prevent future recurrences. This helps to establish a common and agreed understanding or accepted account of what happened, how and why.
Relational approach	Entails the restoration of the social equilibrium through the enactment of social rituals and symbolic acts to help appease the aggrieved party and to re-establish the social order governing the relationship. Strategies include public explanations and apologies, punishment and penance, and compensation to victims.
Regulation and control	Is an effective approach to restore trust among external stakeholders, and when restoring competency-based trust violations in contrast to integrity-based violations and failures. It helps to signal governance intentions and to redefine the boundaries within social relations in the aftermath of trust violations and disrupted social relations.
Ethical culture	Entails repair of trust deficits through a sustained approach wherein organisational routines and procedures are established to promote ethical conduct and to safeguard against unethical behaviour.
Transparency and accountability	Entails the restoration of trust in the aftermath of fraud, and integrity-based violations and failures through approaches that promote 'inward observability' – allowing external stakeholders to monitor the activities and decisions made within the organisation (Grimmelikhuijsen and Meijer, 2014).
Trust transference	This approach to rebuilding trust draws on the argument that trust and distrust can be transferred from one actor or group to another, or from one institutional level (for example, individual, group or system) to another level.

These approaches may need to be applied in combination to achieve the complex task of rebuilding broken trust and relations and also need to be tailored to the local context of institutional and health system governance.

Conclusion: a need for research evidence

This chapter has argued that the erosion of trust in the health system in India is closely tied to the failure of both the regulatory agencies and the professional associations to uphold their mandates. These regulatory failures have been clearly exemplified by the cases of privatisation of medical education; the expansion of the for-profit private provision of health services; and the general failures in implementing and enforcing existing regulations. The chapter considered the relationship between different regulatory approaches and trust relations and outlined the strategic options that might be available for restoring trust. However, there is still limited empirical evidence available on which these policy proposals can be based. Hence, this concluding section identifies possible questions for further research.

It is clear from the analysis presented so far that the evidence available about trust relations in the Indian health care system is in short supply, and so there needs to be a comprehensive study that explores the salience and nature of trust relations in the organisation and practice of stewardship of the Indian health care system, and what shapes these relationships. This would include investigation of the relationship:

- between the state regulatory institutions and those regulated;
- between the various professional bodies and professionals;
- between financing agencies, provider organisations in public and private sectors, and professionals;
- between provider organisations in the public and private sectors, and professionals.

The impact of these chains of trust relations at the institutional and organisational levels on patient and public trust also needs to be explored. Finally, there is a lack of evidence about the effectiveness of different strategies for repairing or restoring trust. The six mechanisms model for restoring and rebuilding trust in institutions outlined in the previous section is a generic model – it needs to be evaluated, specified and validated in the health care-related institutional context, and in the context of different typologies of the governance of health systems.

Notes

[1] Externalities refer to impacts, positive or negative, on individuals or groups who are not involved in a given activity or economic transaction. In the health care context, individuals or groups can benefit from activities undertaken and paid for by others; for example, if a large proportion of children in a community are immunised for certain infectious diseases, the unimmunised children in the community also get protected from infection by virtue of herd immunity. Similarly, individuals and groups can suffer from activities undertaken or not undertaken by others; for example, if individuals with pulmonary tuberculosis do not take timely and appropriate treatment, those in contact with them can get infected. The idea is that health care markets are imperfect because of many instances wherein others can accrue benefits from actions paid for by others, and vice versa.

[2] These unpublished data are taken from an exploratory study carried out by the authors in 2014. For the methodology used in this study, see Kane et al (2015).

References

Arora, R. (2016) 'Becoming a doctor in India: once a cherished dream, no longer cherished though', *Quantitative Imaging in Medicine and Surgery* 6(2): 240-2.

Bachman, R., Gillespie, N. and Priem, R. (2015) 'Repairing trust in organizations and institutions: toward a conceptual framework', *Organization Studies* 36(9): 1123-42.

Baldwin, R. and Black, J. (2008) 'Really responsive regulation', *Modern Law Review* 71(1): 59-94.

Baru, R. (2006) *Privatisation of Health Care in India: A Comparative Analysis of Orissa, Karnataka and Maharashtra States*, CMDR Monograph Series no. 43, Dharwad, India: Centre for Multi-Disciplinary Development Research.

Bloom, G., Kanjilal, B. and Peters, D. (2008) 'Regulating health care markets in China and India', *Health Affairs* 27(4): 952-63.

Bloom, G., Standing, H. and Lloyd, R. (2008) 'Markets, information asymmetry and health care: towards new social contracts', *Social Science and Medicine* 66: 2076-87.

Brown, P. and Calnan, M. (2010) 'The risks of managing uncertainty: the limitations of governance and choice, and the potential for trust', *Social Policy and Society* 9(1): 13-24.

Brown, P. and Calnan, M. (2011) 'The civilizing process of trust: developing quality mechanisms which are local, professional-led and thus legitimate', *Social Policy and Administration* 45(1):19-34.

Brown, P. and Calnan, M. (2016a) 'Chains of (dis)trust: exploring the underpinnings of knowledge sharing and quality care across mental health services', *Sociology of Health and Illness* 38(2): 286-305.

Brown, P. and Calnan, M. (2016b) 'Professionalism, trust and cooperation', in Dent, M., Bourgeault, I. L., Denis, J.-L. and Kuhlmann, E. (eds) *The Routledge Companion to the Professions and Professionalism*, London: Routledge.

Calnan, M. and Rowe, R. (2008) *Trust Matters in Healthcare*, London: Open University Press.

Chatterjee, P. (2010) 'Trouble at the Medical Council of India', *The Lancet* 375: 1679.

D'Cruz, P. and Bharat, S. (2001) 'Which way to turn: inadequacies in the health care system in India', *Journal of Health Management* 3: 85-126.

de Costa, A., Johansson, E. and Diwan, V. (2008) 'Barriers of mistrust: public and private health sectors' perceptions of each other in Madhya Pradesh, India', *Qualitative Health Research* 18(6): 756-66.

Douglass, T. and Calnan, M. (2016) 'Trust matters for doctors; towards an agenda for research', *Social Theory and Health* 14: 393.

Gilson, L., Palmer, N. and Schneider, H. (2005) 'Trust and health worker performance: exploring a conceptual framework using South African evidence', *Social Science and Medicine* 61: 1418-29.

Grimmelikhuijsen, S. J. and Meijer, A. J. (2014) 'The effects of transparency on the perceived trustworthiness of government organization: evidence from an online experiment', *Journal of Public Administration Theory and Research* 24(1): 137-57.

Indian Express (2016) 'Radiologists to go on nationwide strike against PCPNDT Act from September 1', *Indian Express*, 1 September, http://indian express.com/article/india/india-news-india/radiologists-to-go-on-nationwide-strike-against-pcpndt-act-from-september-1/

Indian Medical Association (2016) 'IMA Satyagraha – India Medical Association's open petition', www.ima-india.org/IMASatygraha/

Kane, S., Radkar, A. and Calnan, M. (2015) 'Trust and trust relations from the providers' perspective: the case of the healthcare system in India', *Indian Journal of Medical Ethics* 12(3): 157-68.

Khodyakov, D. (2007) 'Trust as a process', *Sociology* 41(1): 115-32.

Minocha, A. (1980) 'Medical pluralism and health services in India', *Social Science and Medicine* 14(4): 217-23.

Mollering, G. (2001) 'The nature of trust: from Georg Simmel to a theory of expectation, interpretation, and suspension', *Sociology* 35: 403-20.

Nagral, S. (2012) 'Doctors in entrepreneurial gowns', *Economic and Political Weekly* 47(36): 10-12.

Peters, D. H. and Muraleedharan, V. (2008) 'Regulating India's health services: to what end? What future?', *Social Science and Medicine* 66(10): 2133-44.

Phadke, A. (2010) 'The IMA and the Clinical Establishments Act, 2010: irrational opposition to regulation', *Indian Journal of Medical Ethics* 7(4): 229-32.

Phadke, A. (2016) 'Regulation of doctors and private hospitals in India', *Economic and Political Weekly* 6: 46-55.

Pilgrim, D., Tomasini, F. and Yassilev, I. (2010) *Examining Trust in Healthcare: A Multidisciplinary Perspective*, Basingstoke: Palgrave Macmillan.

Rajya Sabha (2016) *The functioning of Medical Council of India*, Report No.92. Rajya Sabha Secretariat, New Delhi: Parliament of India.

Rolfe, A., Cash-Gibson, L., Car, J., Sheikh, A. and McKinstry, B. (2006) 'Interventions for improving patients' trust in doctors and groups of doctors', *Cochrane Database of Systematic Reviews* 3: CD004134.

Sachan, D. (2013) 'Tackling corruption in Indian medicine', *The Lancet* 382: 23-4.

Sen, G. and Iyer, A. (2015) 'Health policy in India: some critical concerns', in Kuhlmann, E., Blank, R. H., Bourgeault, I. L. and Wendt, C. (eds) *The Palgrave International Handbook of Healthcare Policy and Governance*, Basingstoke: Palgrave Macmillan.

Sikri, A. K. (2016) Judgment of the constitutional bench of the Supreme Court of India – Civil Appeal no. 4060 of Modern Dental College and Research Centre and others versus State of Madhya Pradesh and others, 2 May.

Titmuss, R. (2004) 'Choice and the welfare state', in Oakley, A. and Barker, J. (eds) *Private Complaints and Public Health: Richard Titmuss on the NHS*, Bristol: Policy Press.

Tiwari, S. S. (2015) 'Reforming the Medical Council of India', *Indian Journal of Medical Ethics* 12(1): 59.

Vijayakumar, K. and Saini, N. (2013) 'Medical Council of India in a constitutional crisis', *Journal of the Indian Medical Association* 111(10): 706.

Index

Note: Page numbers in *italics* indicate tables. Page numbers followed by n refer to end-of-chapter notes.